Photos of our customers tell you what makes our method different and what it will do for YOU! See our Test of Flexibility Potential (on the last page of this book) to find out if YOU can achieve splits. Follow our method to achieve splits and send us your picture!

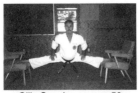

Ollie Speakman, age 50

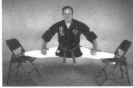

George Dillman, age 51

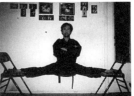

Francisco Hernandez, age 47

"Believe me, I never did full split on the floor or chairs. Look at me at age 47, after 2 months using Mr. Kurz's method."
—Francisco Hernandez

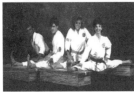

Stephen N. Dileo

"The stretch I have achieved with your techniques has stayed with me despite brief periods of inactivity. This is especially important to me as my schedule sometimes has me traveling where it is impossible to train."
—Stephen N. Dileo

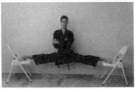

Elias P. Bonaros, Jr.

"After ordering your VHS cassette and book, I have accomplished the impossible! I have been training in the martial arts for 5 years and my flexibility reached a plateau long ago. Now, after using your method for 3 months every day, I have achieved the side split in suspension. In addition, my kicks have become higher and much stronger."
—Elias P. Bonaros

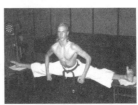

Matt Summers

"I can't believe how well your book works! I have never been able to [do] the full splits or have as much strength as your method has given me. Here is my picture, just so you'll know how well it worked for me. This doesn't even hurt!"
—Matt Summers

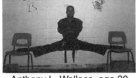

Stephen Dileo's students

"...we [put] your exercises within our class structure and not surprisingly, almost all of our students increased flexibility in a few months."
—Stephen Dileo

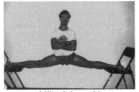

Mike Adrowski

"I have had your book for a couple of years and was able to do the side split after a couple of months. I agree with your statement 'An authority on stretching that can't show this [the split between chairs] is no authority.'"
—Mike Adrowski

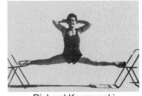

Richard Korczynski

"My legs are strong and I was fairly flexible, but I got stuck one foot above the ground in a split. Now I do it on chairs after using your method for only one month."
—Richard Korczynski

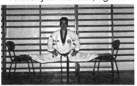

Anthony L. Wallace, age 30

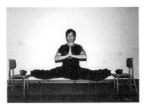

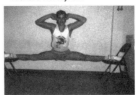

Piotr Stabinski

David Cruz, age 30

Dave Walk

Testimonials

"In the last two months my flexibility has improved more than in six years of [stretching in a] gym"—Marcello Clarizia, Rome, Italy

"I could feel it from the first day. Unbelievable!"—Marwan Hassanein, Risskov, Denmark

"My range of flexibility and more importantly, the looseness and agility of my muscles improved ten times faster than with any of the other 'experts' methods. My classmates are in awe of the fact that I can be warmed up and ready to work out in about five minutes, and that I can kick well over my head without a warm-up."
—Donny L. Ables, Jr., Tyler, Texas

"The book and video have been a great value for me personally, but I also treat athletes from a variety of backgrounds and I encourage them to buy your products as well"—Dr. Martin P. Marcus, Marcus Chiropractic Clinic, St. Petersburg, Florida

"... I have never been able to display my maximum range of motion without thoroughly warming up, a process lasting some 30 to 45 minutes, and muscles would always be limited in mobility early in the morning. Using your method, I am able to achieve the same stretch in only five minutes, and perform with maximal range of motion even in the morning! ...stretching is no longer a tedious task. Stretching Scientifically is, without doubt, the most effective, efficient and safest method of stretching..."—H. D. Palfrey, karate instructor, Gillingham, England

"Prior to buying your book I had spent long periods using traditional type stretching, i.e., sitting on the floor in a 'box split position' stretching from side to side (none bounce). Before kicking I had to spend 20 to 30 minutes stretching. This I had to do 2 or 3 times a day. Using your method this situation has improved. Now after warming up and leg lifts I can kick reasonably well."—M. Richardson, karate instructor, Stafford, Staffordshire, England

"Your book has given me a new life in taekwondo. Before I got the book I would have to go down to the gym 45 min. before the black belt class, but now it takes 15 min. to warm up. I have not had one injury since I got the book."—Thomas R. Phoenix, Jr., taekwondo instructor, Republic of Ireland

"Your book Stretching Scientifically is excellent. It gives the scientific basis for your techniques and then a good description of each exercise."—Steven Gerrish, university professor, Sault Ste. Marie, Michigan

"I have been applying your Stretching Scientifically for some time. My fellow taekwon-doists noticed a difference in my flexibility almost right away! I can do a split in suspension now, and am working on my split with toes pointing upward. With your method, I hope to achieve this split this year!"—Marco E. Castañeda, Quito, Equador

"You explain better and prove it [effectiveness of your method]"—Julian Ingerson, Tinley Park, Illinois

"I felt results on the first day of [using] Stretching Scientifically. My kicks are much higher and stronger now"—August A. Guadamuz, San Carlos, California

"While reading and almost instantly, I made improvements in my kicking. Can't wait to finish. I get better stretch, plus knowledge as to why a particular movement is necessary"—Ralph Velazquez, Brooklyn, New York

"An outstanding book. I get closer to my goal of a full split almost every time I stretch"—Thomas Hawthorne, police officer, Exeter, New Hampshire

Stretching Scientifically

A Guide to Flexibility Training

Fourth edition

by Thomas Kurz

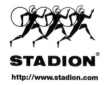

STADION®

http://www.stadion.com

Thomas Kurz—athlete, p.e. teacher, and coach—studied at Akademia Wychowania Fizycznego (University School of Physical Education) in Warsaw, Poland. His knowledge of both the coach's and athlete's perspective gives the reader of *Stretching Scientifically* a full-spectrum survey of the best information available. His other highly regarded work is the *Science of Sports Training: How to Plan and Control Training for Peak Performance*. He also translated and edited Prof. Józef Drabik's *Children and Sports Training*, and coach Tadeusz Starzynski's and Prof. Henryk Sozanski's *Explosive Power and Jumping Ability for All Sports*.

Published by:

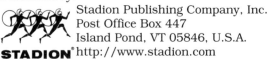 Stadion Publishing Company, Inc.
Post Office Box 447
Island Pond, VT 05846, U.S.A.
STADION http://www.stadion.com

Copyright © 1987, 1990, 1991, 1994, 2003 by Thomas Kurz
Printed in the United States of America

Publisher's Cataloging-in-Publication
(Provided by Quality Books, Inc.)

Kurz, Thomas, 1956-
    Stretching scientifically : a guide to flexibility
training / by Thomas Kurz. — 4th ed.
    p. cm.
    Includes bibliographical references and index.
    LCCN 2002096216
    ISBN 0-940149-45-1

    1. Physical education and training. 2. Physical
fitness. 3. Stretching exercises. I. Title.

GV711.5.K87 2003   613.7'1
                              QBI02-200946

Editing by R. Scott Perry
Cover Design by TLC Graphics © 2003, www.TLCGraphics.com
Cover Photo by Chuck Shahood
Book Design by Eva Chodkiewicz-Swider
Drawings by Eva Chodkiewicz-Swider
Photography by Chuck Shahood and Don Whipple

I dedicate this book to the late Antoni Zagorski and the late Tadeusz Sadowski. Without their help it would have never been written.

Warning—Disclaimer

The author and Stadion Publishing Company are not liable or responsible to any person or entity for any damage caused or alleged to be caused directly or indirectly by the information contained in this book.

Consult your physician before starting any exercise program.

Due to the rapid increase of range of motion some martial artists experience while using this method of flexibility training, they may kick higher than they are used to and miss their targets. With a little practice, however, they will regain their accuracy.

Whenever there are particular cautions for you to observe, they are signaled for you like this:

> Caution: Pick only one isometric stretch per muscle group and repeat it two to five times, using as many tensions per repetition as it takes to reach the limit of mobility that you now have.

TABLE OF CONTENTS

Preface

In this book you will find all the information about flexibility training you may need for your sport.

My first book on this subject, published in 1985, was a great success. Several readers wrote me about the gains they had made thanks to my instruction. There were readers, though, who had difficulty understanding these instructions because of their preconceptions about training. Others after initial rapid gains reached a level well short of their goal (and their potential) and could not progress any further. Using the feedback from all these readers, in this, the fourth edition, I have completely reorganized the book and rewritten parts to make it even more understandable and more informative.

If you have read only the books and research papers on flexibility that were published in what used to be called the West (North America and the noncommunist countries of Europe), you will notice that I sometimes use different terms in writing about this subject. Other times familiar terms may denote something different than the meaning you are used to. This is so because I was trained in a completely different system of physical education and sports. The terms I use are a direct translation of the terms used in the former East bloc's physical education and sports training methods.

With the collapse of the Soviet Union, the term *East bloc* is rapidly assuming a status of quaint antiquity. It was used to refer to the nations of Eastern Europe that had been unwillingly absorbed by the U.S.S.R. For decades these nations—especially Poland, East Germany, Hungary, and Rumania—dominated Olympic and other international athletic contests far beyond what one might expect based on size and resources. The difference lay in their common use of advanced methods of training.

The Methodology of P.E. and Sports is the central subject in university courses for coaches and P.E. teachers there. It is a body of knowledge that makes all the difference between success and failure in developing athletic skills and abilities, or simply in getting results from one's exercises. In describing the methods of stretching, I have given as much information about the correct ways of working out as possible without making this book a complete manual on the methodology of physical education and sports training. To do so would make this book unwieldy and would duplicate information contained in *Science of Sports Training: How to Plan and Control Training for Peak Performance*, another work available through Stadion Publishing.

Acknowledgments

Everything I know about physical education, sports, and training, I have learned from teachers at Akademia Wychowania Fizycznego (Academy of Physical Education). They taught me the most modern (if something so advanced can be called merely modern) methods of training. To them, and all East European P.E. teachers and coaches, this book is nothing new, because all I did was put in writing what they have been teaching for many years. I am especially grateful to my teachers for bringing the importance of methodology of physical education and sports to the attention of me and my fellow students.

Introduction
Getting the Most Out of This Book

The essence of flexibility training presented in this book is the simultaneous development of strength and flexibility, working with your body (especially the nervous system), for full flexibility with no warm-up.

The method of accomplishing these goals can be summed up in a single paragraph: Tense your muscles prior to relaxing and stretching them, and tense them every time when you want to increase your range of motion during a stretch. To simultaneously develop strength and flexibility, tense your muscles while they are fully stretched. As your strength in stretched positions increases, so does your range of motion and your ability to use increasingly greater range of motion without a warm-up. To develop the ability to instantaneously show full flexibility in dynamic movements, do dynamic stretches (such as arm or leg swings) for a few minutes twice every day. That is all. The rest are details, but these details make all the difference between effective training and fruitless drudgery. That is what the rest of this book is about.

How to use this book

This book gives you all the information you need to accomplish the maximum flexibility permitted by the bone structure of your joints and by their ligaments. You will be able to display your increased flexibility without any warm-up in both dynamic movements such as kicks and in static positions such as splits.

Read chapter 1, "Flexibility in Sports," for fundamental information about the kinds of flexibility. Think of it as the basic definitions you need to know. In addition you will find key principles regarding

1

injury prevention and some cautions about possible causes of difficulties you may encounter.

You will find many exercises here, but you need only a few of them to gain all the flexibility you need for your sport. Which exercises you need depends mainly on your sport and on your personal characteristics.

If you are a gymnast you need all types of flexibility, so you will select needed exercises from chapters 3 ("Dynamic Stretching"), 4 ("Static Active Stretching"), 5 ("Isometric Stretching"), and 6 ("Relaxed Stretching").

If you are a karateka, kickboxer, taekwondo player, or an athlete of any combat sport that calls for full-extension kicks, you will select from among the exercises shown in chapters 3 ("Dynamic Stretching"), 5 ("Isometric Stretching"), and 6 ("Relaxed Stretching").

If you are a swimmer or track-and-field athlete you will select exercises from chapters 3 ("Dynamic Stretching"), 5 ("Isometric Stretching"), and 6 ("Relaxed Stretching").

If you are a wrestler (Greco-Roman, free-style, judo, sambo, or other), you will need exercises mainly from chapters 5 ("Isometric Stretching") and 6 ("Relaxed Stretching"). If your technique calls for great dynamic flexibility of the legs, such as the inner thigh rip of judo and other styles of jacket wrestling, you will also need one or more exercises from chapter 3 ("Dynamic Stretching").

No matter what sport you participate in, you should read chapter 2, "How to Stretch." It tells when to do which exercises and how to arrange them in any single workout. Chapter 7, "Sample Workout Plans," shows how to apply the principles of arranging the exercises in practice. These examples are not for slavish imitation but to illustrate a rational selection and flow of exercises.

Chapter 8, "All the Whys of Stretching," will give you a full understanding of this method of flexibility training. Knowing the theory, why the exercises are to be done in some particular way and what their effect is on the body, helps with designing training programs.

Chapter 9 of the book, "Questions and Answers on Stretching," consists of typical questions on flexibility training from athletes. If you read the whole book you will know answers to nearly all these questions, in which case the content of this chapter will serve primarily for your amusement.

1. Flexibility in Sports

There are six kinds of flexibility, with classification depending on the character of the muscles' action and on the presence or absence of an external force that aids moving through the range of motion or assuming and maintaining a stretched position (Tumanyan and Kharatsidis 1998). These six kinds are:

- dynamic active flexibility (only using the muscles of the moving body part);

- dynamic passive flexibility below the pain threshold (using as much external assistance as needed to reach the painless limit of motion);

- dynamic passive flexibility over the pain threshold and up to pain tolerance (using as much external assistance as needed to reach the maximal limit of motion permitted by pain tolerance);

- static active flexibility (only using the muscles of the stretched body part to hold a stretched position);

- static passive flexibility below the pain threshold (using as much external assistance as needed to reach the painless maximum stretch); and

- static passive flexibility up to pain tolerance (using as much external assistance as needed to reach the maximal stretch permitted by pain tolerance).

Practically speaking, however, in training practice usually three kinds of flexibility are deliberately developed—dynamic active, static active, and static passive (below the pain threshold).

3

Dynamic active flexibility. This is the ability to perform dynamic movements within a full range of motion in the joints. It is best developed by dynamic stretching. This kind of flexibility depends on the ability to combine relaxation of the extended muscles with contraction of the moving muscles.

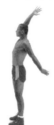
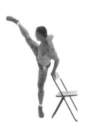

Examples of dynamic active flexibility

Static active flexibility. This is the ability to assume and maintain extended positions using only the tension of the agonists and synergists while the antagonists are being stretched. One example is lifting the leg and keeping it high without any support. An athlete's static active flexibility depends on the athlete's static passive flexibility and on the static strength of the muscles that stabilize the position.

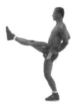

Examples of static active flexibility

Static passive flexibility. This is the ability to assume and maintain extended positions using your weight (splits), or using strength not coming from the stretched limbs, such as lifting and holding a leg with your arm or by other external means.

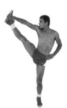

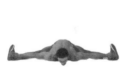

Examples of static passive flexibility

Passive flexibility usually exceeds active (static and dynamic) flexibility in the same joint. The greater this difference, the greater the flexibility reserve and the greater the possibility of increasing the amplitude of active movements. This difference diminishes in training as active flexibility improves. Doing static stretching alone does not guarantee an increase of dynamic flexibility proportional to the increase of static flexibility (Matveyev [Matveev] 1981).

The principles of flexibility training are the same in all sports. Only the required level of a given kind of flexibility varies from sport to sport.

The flexibility of an athlete is sufficiently developed when the maximal reach of motion somewhat exceeds the reach required in competition. This difference between an athlete's flexibility and the needs of the sport is called "the flexibility reserve" or "tensility reserve." It allows the athlete to do techniques without excessive tension and prevents injury. Achieving the maximum speed in an exercise is impossible at your extreme ranges of motion, i.e., when you have no "flexibility reserve."

The training of flexibility, as well as of any other motor ability, should proceed in form from general to sport-specific—reflecting the needs of particular sports. In choosing stretches, you should examine your needs and the requirements of your activity. For example, if you are a hurdler, you need mostly a dynamic flexibility of hips, trunk, and shoulders. To increase your range of motion, you need to do dynamic leg raises in all directions, bends and twists of the trunk, and arm swings. You can perfect your technique by doing various dynamic exercises consisting of walking or running over the hurdles. The hurdler's stretch, a static exercise, does not fit into your workout because it strains your knee by twisting it. Simple front and side splits are better for stretching your legs. The explanation that in the hurdler's stretch your position resembles the one assumed while passing the hurdle is pointless. You cannot learn dynamic skills by using static exercises, and vice versa. The technique of running over the hurdles is better developed in motion.

In karate or kickboxing, punches, blows, and kicks should hit their targets with maximum speed. Some targets require nearly fully stretched muscles of the hitting limb (in the case of kicks, also of the supporting leg). Your nervous system has a way of making sure that a stretch, particularly a sudden one, does not end abruptly, causing a muscle tear. But a gradual slowing down before the moment of contact will spoil the impact. Therefore, you have to train your nervous system so you can have maximal speed at the moment of contact even if it is close to the maximal reach of motion in this movement. In the case of kicks, you can learn this skill by using your hand as a target for them. Centers in your brain that regulate coordination and rapid movements know about the hand. They know where it is and that it can stop the kick, so the leg does not have to be slowed down gradually to prevent overstretching.

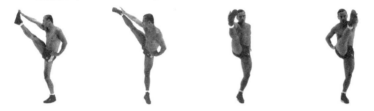

Examples of exercises developing the ability to kick with maximum speed at the ranges of motion required in fighting

You must first develop the ability to move your limbs with moderate speed within a full range of motion in joints in order to do these specific kicking drills. You should start at a lower height to avoid injury from any sudden contraction of rapidly stretched muscles. You can use this exercise only in a warm-up because of the limited variety of kicks that you can practice this way.

Fighters relying on high kicks as their combat techniques should spend a few minutes in the morning on the dynamic stretching of their legs. Starting slowly, they should gradually raise the legs higher. Later they should increase the speed of their movements, perhaps even using the previously described "hand-kicking" drill. Practical experience (North Korean, Soviet bloc's commando units) shows that doing the actual combat kicks in this morning stretch is not necessary to be able to do them later in a day without a warm-up.

Wrestlers (freestyle, Greco-Roman, judo, and others) need especially great static strength in extreme ranges of motion to get out of holds and locks. They will best develop this strength by isometric stretching and lifting weights through the full range of motion along appropriate paths.

Gymnasts and acrobats must display a high degree of development of all kinds of flexibility, with greater emphasis on static active flexibility than in any other sport. Training for and displaying static active flexibility requires good strength in the trunk muscles, especially in the lower back.

Rowers should have hamstrings long enough to allow them to lean far forward at the catch phase of the rowing stroke without flexing the lumbar spine much. If the hamstrings are short, the rowers compensate by flexing the spine more than 50% of its maximum range of flexion. Such flexing, combined with the high compressive and shearing forces acting on the spine during rowing, contributes to hyperflexion of the spine—which correlates strongly with low back pain (Reid and McNair 2000; Howell 1984).

Swimmers should have long hamstrings and chest muscles. When doing the breaststroke, if you go up and down in the water instead of moving just under the surface, it means that your chest muscles are too short. In the backstroke this shortness also causes your face to submerge when the arm enters the water, which is when you want to take a breath. In the crawl, short hamstrings pull your feet out of the water and make your legwork inefficient. Poor flexibility of ankles and toes makes a swimmer ride low in the water. (Ankle flexibility can be improved by wearing fins while doing kick sets, and toe extensions and curls improve flexibility and strength of the toes.)

You should be careful in choosing your stretches, however, because too much flexibility in some parts of the body can be detrimental to your sports performance or just unhealthy. For example, even though swimmers need more than a normal range of motion in the shoulders, their internal rotators' stretches should not go beyond the frontal plane of the body to avoid damaging the joint capsule and cartilage at the front of shoulder joint, which would lead to shoulder instability (Bak and Magnusson 1997). Forced stretching—past the point where you can move using the stretched muscles—can damage the capsule of the shoulder joint, leading to shoulder instability and pain (McMaster and Troup 1993; McMaster et al. 1998). Female gymnasts with symptoms of musculoskeletal disorders of the lower back can touch the floor behind their feet in a standing position farther than those without symptoms (Kirby et al. 1981). This may be caused by having weak or overstretched (inhibited by excessive stretching) hamstrings or muscles of the buttocks (Walther 2000). Another possible cause of the low back discomfort, in gymnasts who can touch the floor very far behind their heels in a standing position, could be poor form in performing stretches for lumbar flexion, such as the toe-touching stretches— rounding the back when leaning forward. During such stretches the spine should be kept "straight"—with its normal, natural curves just like when you are standing upright—so the movement occurs mainly in the hip joints. Rounding the lower back can overstretch its muscles and ligaments and cause a lifetime of back pain (Alter 1996).

Some Olympic weightlifters may need to tighten the muscles surrounding the hip and knee joints for the proper execution of lifts. Muscles that are too relaxed at long length let the weightlifter "sink" too deep on the legs while getting under the barbell. This makes it difficult to stand up and complete the lift.

Running economy has been associated with decreased flexibility. Stiffness of the calf muscles and Achilles tendon enhances "elastic energy storage and return" during every running step, and the small range of motion of external rotation in the hip reduces the metabolic cost of the muscular activity needed for stabilizing the pelvis during long-distance running (Craib et al. 1996). Excessive mobility in the joints diminishes stability of the body, causing scattering of the forces acting on it. This in turn necessitates additional muscular tension in movements where parts of the body have to be stabilized to support heavy loads (Raczek 1991). Such scattering of forces—for example, caused by an excessively loose trunk at the moment of takeoff—reduces performance in jumping (Wazny 1981b).

Maximal force production in bench press, one of the events of powerlifting, is positively related to the stiffness of prime movers if the bench press is done without a rebound (Wilson et al. 1994), so flexibility training could affect it adversely, but performance in a bench press done with a rebound benefits from flexibility training (Wilson et al. 1992). Performance in sprint (a speed-strength effort) improved when both weight training and stretching were included with sprint training as compared to sprint training alone (Dintiman 1964). At the very least Dintiman's experiment showed that adding stretching to sprint training did not lower the running speed.

To take advantage of a rebound, the stiffer the muscles and tendons the better, provided you have the required range of motion (Kubo et al. 1999). If your range of motion is less than required for full utilization of the rebound, then high stiffness does not help and it may be economical to increase range of motion, even at the cost of lowering somewhat the stiffness of your involved muscles and tendons (Wilson et al. 1992).

Having muscles so short and stiff they limit the range of motion required in your sport may cause an overuse injury (Krivickas 1997; Howell 1984).

Saxton and Donnelly (1996) showed that resistance exercises consisting of eccentric muscle actions (in which muscles tense as they are being stretched) caused loss of strength at short muscle length. According to them this loss of strength at short length suggests that an increase in muscle length has occurred, perhaps due to elongation of the sarcomeres, or elongation of connective tissue of the muscle and tendon, or both.

Injury prevention and flexibility

Whether high or low flexibility prevents or predisposes for injuries in sports depends on the sport and on the athlete's favorite techniques. In some sports, poor flexibility in some movements may cause overuse injuries, while in others, a less than average flexibility improves performance. Here is what Gleim and McHugh (1997) say.

"It is possible that flexibility patterns which represent risk factor for one sport may not do so for another. . . . No clear relationship can be described between flexibility and injury that is applicable to all sports and levels of play. While increased flexibility is important for performance in some sports that rely on extremes of motion for movement, decreased flexibility may actually increase economy of movement in sports which use only the midportion of range of movement" (Gleim and McHugh 1997).

> Most muscle strains "are believed to occur during eccentric contractions, which can cause damage within the normal range of motion. . . . If injuries usually occur within the normal range of motion, why would an increased range of motion prevent injuries?" (Shrier 2000).

A muscle does not have to be maximally stretched to be torn. Muscle tears are the result of a special combination of a stretch and a contraction at the same time (Garrett 1996), and neither the stretch nor the contraction has to be maximal. Sometimes the contraction is really a spasm, resulting from a chronic weakness of the muscle. Even the most flexible athlete can develop an overuse injury that manifests itself as a muscle spasm. If the athlete continues to exercise with a muscle spasm, eventually a strong tension of the affected muscle may (and often does) tear it. So you see that great flexibility alone will not prevent injuries. Actually, excessive development of flexibility leads to irreversible deformation of the joints, which distorts posture and adversely affects performance (Matveyev [Matveev] 1981). For example, repeated forceful hyperextensions of the back may damage vertebra in adolescents (Harvey and Tanner 1991). In baseball and swimming, laxity of the glenohumeral joint predisposes the joint for injuries (Fleisig et al. 1995; McMaster et al. 1998; Pappas et al. 1985).

> Low back pain may result from laxity of joints other than those of the back—lax ligaments of ankle and knee joints increase the risk of low back pain (Nadler et al. 1998). You can compensate for lax ligaments by strengthening the muscles crossing a given joint (Krivickas 1997; Zelisko et al. 1982).

There are four main causes of injuries: great differences in strength between two opposing muscle groups; strength and flexibility imbalances between the same muscle groups on both sides of the body; a difference of fatigability (muscle endurance) between the limbs; and imbalances in activity of muscles (Burkett 1970; Knapik et al. 1991; Murphy 1991; Orchard et al. 1997; McMaster et al. 1991; Rudy 1987; Tyler et al. 2001). According to Murphy (1991) imbalances in activity are more likely to cause an injury than imbalances in strength.

> Differences in strength of the same muscle groups on both sides of the body, when measured at a given velocity, should not exceed 10 percent (Feiring and Derscheid 1989).

More specific information on the proper ratios of strength among muscle groups is in *Science of Sports Training: How to Plan and Control Training for Peak Performance.*

Unbalanced flexibility, i.e., an abnormally large range of motion in some movements but less than normal in other movements in the same joint, may contribute to injuries. In classical ballet, where dancers have an extraordinary range of external rotation and abduction of the hip combined with less than normal internal rotation and adduction, 30% of dancers complain of lateral knee pain and 33% of anterior hip pain (Reid et al. 1987). In nonathletic people, a range of external rotation in the hips greater by more than 10 degrees than the range of internal rotation is associated with low back pain (Ellison et al. 1990). So, for safety's sake, do some stretches in directions that are not typical for your sport or at least do some of your stretches in the full range of motion. For example, do leg swings from full adduction (across your body) to full abduction or arm rotations from full external rotation to full internal rotation.

Balancing the flexibility of all the muscles in a joint and improving the strength and endurance of the weaker muscles are the easiest measures for prevention of injuries. A careful analysis of your form of movement may also hold the key to injury prevention. A good technique feels effortless. Eliminate those moments in your technique in which you use the maximal tension of already stretched muscles to counter the fast movement of a relatively big mass. Such movements may lead to tears in the muscles of a supporting leg in kicking, for example. Likewise, if you abruptly strain against great external resistance, or against the inertia of your body, it may lead to a muscle strain—for example, a hamstring tear in starting a sprint from the starting blocks.

If one muscle group, or muscles of one limb or one side of the body are more tensed than other muscles, you may have a nerve problem or misaligned bones. For example, a twisted pelvis will cause one hamstring to be more tensed than the other. Stretching overly tensed muscles cannot fix the cause of their abnormal tension. In this example, it neither realigns the pelvis nor addresses the cause of this misalignment, which can be neurological or mechanical. While stretching may temporarily make you feel better, it will not remove the threat of potential injury. This is why static stretching before working out does not prevent injuries. Research bears this out—the majority of studies show static stretches before working out to be detrimental or of no benefit for injury prevention (Shrier 2000). Pre-exercise static stretching does not prevent soreness, tenderness, or the force loss that follows eccentric exercise (Johansson et al. 1999).

In instances of excessive tension (excessive neural stimulation) or weakness (excessive neural inhibition) caused by misaligned joints or neurological problems, typical strength training exercises will not help you either. Typical strength exercises will either overstress the overly tensed muscles or will bypass the weak ones by recruiting others to do their job. To fix such problems you need the help of an *applied kinesiology*[1] specialist who, among other modes

---

1   Applied kinesiology is a science of human movement, human structure, and the biochemistry of nutrition. *Kinesiology* means the knowledge of body motion, especially muscle function, and how it relates to the rest of the body systems. *Applied* refers to

of treatment, may prescribe special exercises for normalizing the tension of muscles.

The fact that static stretching, or any strenuous stretching, right before exercising is useless or even harmful does not mean that you may not stretch strenuously at all. Just do it after the other exercises. In the case of exercises that do considerable damage to the muscles, such as very hard resistance exercises, do stretches several hours later. Stretching during the acute phase of muscle damage would compound the damage. Even static stretching can put enough stress on the muscle fibers to damage them. For persons just beginning a workout program, stretching alone—either ballistic or static—may cause delayed onset muscle soreness, which is a symptom of muscle damage (Smith et al. 1993).

This is a how-to-do-it book about stretching, but you needed to know a little why-to-do-it before you got started. Now you are ready to begin.

---

putting this knowledge to practical use. Applied kinesiology uses very specific muscle testing, gait and posture analysis, blood and urine testing, and other noninvasive, inexpensive diagnostic methods. Once a diagnosis is made, therapy may include spinal, cranial, and extremity manipulation (adjustment of joints in the back, neck, skull, and in limbs), myofascial therapies, muscle stimulation, special exercises, as well as changes in diet. Addresses of applied kinesiologists are available from the International College of Applied Kinesiology, Web site http://www.icak.com.

2. How to Stretch

The right stretching method will let you have great flexibility even without a warm-up. Such flexibility is essential for coaches so they can demonstrate a technique immediately when it is needed. A lack of this ability indicates either that the stretching method you use is incorrect, you are chronically fatigued, or both.

> Caution: In spite of having this ability you should not abuse it. It is fine to do a few full range-of-motion moves without warm-up, but not many. Take kickboxing or karate kicks, for example— kicks involve sudden twisting or bending of the trunk, so not warming up can result in back pain. The back is wrapped in deep layers of muscles, and the larger and deeper the mass of muscles, the more time it takes to warm it up. Warming up before effort facilitates recovery after it.

Developing great flexibility is one of the easiest tasks in athletic training. It takes little time and effort to reach an exceptional level. With rational training flexibility improves from day to day (Ozolin 1971). Why then do so many people spend hours weekly, year after year, and get such meager results? Here are the most common causes of difficulties in developing athletic form, flexibility in particular.

The wrong warm-up. Doing static stretches does not sufficiently raise muscle temperature, it does not increase blood flow through muscles, it does not warm up joints, or prepare you for further effort.

The wrong training load. Training loads that are too great without enough rest cause chronic fatigue. If you begin your workout still sore after the previous one, you are asking for an injury or at least you hamper your further progress.

The wrong sequence of efforts. If you use the wrong sequence of efforts in a workout or in a microcycle, it may double or triple your recovery time. (A microcycle is a set of workouts. It usually lasts one week. Information on how to arrange workouts in microcycles is in *Science of Sports Training: How to Plan and Control Training for Peak Performance.*)

The wrong methods. Incorrect methods of teaching skills may result in too many repetitions of a given exercise and chronic local fatigue. Choosing methods that develop athletic abilities and skills in ways that interfere with the development of flexibility as well as total athletic development is really an umbrella difficulty that covers all the problems.

Applying the methodology you find advocated here in your training will prevent you from making any of the preceding mistakes. These principles are included in the descriptions of stretching methods. If you follow the instructions to the letter, you will not go wrong.

Methods of stretching

There are several methods for improving flexibility. In this book you will find only the safest and most efficient of these. Your choice of method (or combination of methods) depends on your sport and the shape you are in.

Dynamic stretching. Dynamic stretching involves moving parts of your body and gradually increasing reach, speed of movement, or both. Perform your exercises (for instance, leg raises or arm swings) in sets of eight to twelve repetitions. If after a few sets you feel tired—stop. Fatigue causes a decrease in the amplitude of your movements. Do only the number of repetitions that you can do without diminishing your range of motion. More repetitions will only set the nervous regulation of the muscles' length at the level of these less than best repetitions and may cause you to lose some of your flexibility. What you repeat more times or with a greater effort will leave a deeper trace in your memory! After reaching the maximal range of motion in a joint in any direction of movement, you should not do many more repetitions of this movement in a given workout. Even if you can maintain your current maximal range of motion over many repetitions, you will set an unnecessarily solid memory of the range of these movements. You will then have to overcome these memories in order to make further progress.

Dynamic stretches do not involve stopping and holding the stretched position. Such holding is the feature of static active stretches (see definition below on this page).

One relatively recent study (Bandy et al. 1998) confuses the issue somewhat by misnaming certain static active stretches as "dynamic range of motion exercises." A reader misled by that term, which Bandy applies to raise-and-hold stretches, might wrongly conclude that dynamic stretching doesn't measure up to what it is supposed to do.

What is dynamic stretching supposed to do? It increases dynamic active flexibility. Your body in motion increases its speed of movement, or its range, or both. These are results you measure in dynamic motions, not in static positions.

Do not confuse dynamic stretching with ballistic stretching either. In ballistic stretches, you use the momentum of a fast-moving body or a limb to forcibly and abruptly increase the range of motion. Ballistic movement cannot be adjusted or corrected once started. Ballistic or bounce stretches may result in immediate as well as residual pain—the symptom of "minute injury to soft tissue involved in the stretching," which the subsequent strenuous exercises may aggravate" to the point of serious muscle damage" (Logan and Egstrom 1961). Nelson and Kokkonen (2001) showed that maximal force in knee flexion declined on the average by 7.5% and in knee extension by 5.6% after six 15-second ballistic stretches—bobbing in a stretch—even though more than 10 minutes passed between ballistic stretching and strength tests.

In dynamic stretching (as opposed to ballistic stretching) there are no bobbing, bouncing, or jerky movements and the movements are controlled thoroughly even though they are quite fast. In dynamic stretching the stretch is not sudden, unlike in ballistic stretching.

Practically, the same dynamic stretch (for example, a leg swing) can be performed with control through the whole range of movement or with no control over a substantial part of the movement when the stretch takes place, or as anything in between.

Static active stretching. Static active stretching involves moving your body into a stretch and holding it there through the tension of the muscle-agonists in this movement. You may notice that the harder you tense the agonistic muscles the less resistance you feel from the stretched muscles.

Static active stretches increase both your static active range of motion and your static passive range of motion (Bandy et al. 1998; Roberts and Wilson 1999). Longer (15 seconds) static active stretches are more effective for increasing an active range of motion than shorter (5 seconds) ones. Both durations (5 seconds and 15 seconds) cause similar increases in the passive range of motion— which exceed the static active range (Roberts and Wilson 1999).

Relaxed stretching for static passive flexibility. Relaxed stretching involves relaxing your body into a stretch and holding it there by the weight of your body or by some other external force. This type of stretching is more effective than dynamic stretching for increasing the static passive range of motion and decreasing the amount of force needed to hold a stretch—the tension in a static position (McNair and Stanley 1996; McNair et al. 2001). Relaxed stretches increase static passive range of motion more than static active stretches (Bandy et al. 1998).

like both physios

Relaxed stretches relieve cramps of overstimulated muscles. Slow and light relaxed static stretching is useful in relieving spasms occurring in muscles that are healing after an injury or are just sore (deVries 1961). Stretching of sore muscles, however, may further damage them. After all, soreness is a sign of muscle tissue damage and Smith et al. (1993) showed that stretching may cause delayed onset muscle soreness. So, if you feel that a stretch may relieve spasms in the sore muscles, to be safe stretch lightly—only as much as it takes to feel relief.

> Caution: After an injury you should not exercise or stretch at all until you have healed sufficiently and you have checked it with your doctor.

For increasing static range of motion the most effective duration of relaxed stretches is 30 seconds, and the most effective frequency is once per day (Bandy and Irion 1994; Bandy et al. 1997).

Like Jamie's example.

Isometric stretching for static passive flexibility. Using positions similar to those in static passive stretching and adding the strong tensions of stretched muscles, you can cause postcontractive relaxations and, subsequently, increases in the stretch.[1] For a greater effect as you relax the stretched muscle, you can tense its

---

[1]   These relaxations following strong tensions feel just like Dr. Jacobson's Progressive Relaxation.

antagonists, i.e., the muscles that oppose it (Etnyre and Abraham 1986a). Eventually, when you achieve your maximal (at this stage of training) stretch, you hold the last tension for several seconds. This increases the strength of the muscles in this position. Even without these last tensions, contract-relax stretching improves your range of motion both in passive and active movements as well as your strength in concentric, isometric, and especially in eccentric actions (Handel et al. 1997).

Isometric stretching is the fastest and the most efficient method of increasing static passive range of motion (Etnyre and Abraham 1986a; Holt et al. 1970; Lucas and Koslow 1984; Sady et al. 1982; Tanigawa 1972). Because of the strong and long tensions in this type of stretching, apply it according to the same principles as other strength exercises. You should allow sufficient time for recovery after exercising, depending on your shape and on the total volume of exercises, their intensity, and the sequence of efforts. Do not exercise so hard as to make your muscles sore and do not exercise sore muscles strenuously. Muscle soreness is accompanied by loss of strength and of range of motion (Miles and Clarkson 1994), so if you make your muscles sore often you will reduce your flexibility. Muscle shortening is most pronounced 2 days after performing the exercises that caused muscle soreness (Clarkson et al. 1992). It is a good idea to do isometric stretches in strength workouts and, on days when recovering from these workouts, do either static relaxed stretches or replace the last, long tension in your isometric stretches by just holding the relaxed muscles in the final stretch.

To increase static passive flexibility do isometric stretches at least twice a week, depending on your recovery, though. Wallin et al. (1985) recommends isometric or contract-relax stretching from three to five times a week. The best time for isometric stretching is the end of a workout—this is the time when isometric stretches are most effective (Moller et al. 1985). For maintaining flexibility it may be enough to do isometric (contract-relax) stretching once per week (Wallin et al. 1985). You will get help in sorting these varying recommendations in chapter 5.

Doing both isometric and static active stretching, you will most quickly develop static forms of flexibility.

To develop passive mobility up to 90% of what is anatomically possible, for ankle and knee joints it usually takes up to 30 days; for joints of the spine, up to 60 days; and for hip joints, from 60 to 120 days (Starzynski and Sozanski 1999).

Tumanyan and Dzhanyan (1980) in their research on passive and active forms of static flexibility showed that:

—passive stretching, which increases passive range of motion, causes parallel increases in active range of motion with the difference between them unchanged;

—strength exercises done throughout the full range of motion increase active range of motion and so reduce the difference between passive and active range of motion; and

—doing both passive stretching and strength exercises increases both passive and active range of motion while decreasing the difference between them.

Strength exercises for increasing flexibility are similar to stretches, except that what would be the final position of a stretch is the initial position of a strength exercise. For example, strength exercises for increasing shoulder flexibility are done from stretched positions, with resistance light enough to stretch the exercised muscles without the danger of overstretching them (Platonov 1997; Platonov and Fesenko 1990). Making 3- to 5-second stops at the maximal stretch increases the effectiveness of these exercises (Platonov 1997). When the resistance is just right (not too heavy), the range of motion increases in each successive set of such exercises. If the strength exercises merely involve all muscles around a joint but do not put them on a stretch in every possible direction, they may cause loss of flexibility in the unexercised directions (Girouard and Hurley 1995).

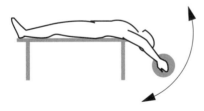

Strength exercise for increasing flexibility

Early morning stretching

If you need to perform movements requiring considerable flexibility with no warm-up, you ought to make the early morning stretch a part of your daily routine (Ozolin 1971; Wazny 1981b). Early morning stretching, which you would do before breakfast, consists of a few sets of dynamic movements—for example, arm swings and leg raises to the front, rear, and sides. Before doing these dynamic stretches, warm up all your joints with easy movements. Do the stretching before breakfast because after the meal blood flow in the muscles is diminished, which decreases flexibility, and because doing dynamic stretches, such as high leg raises, with a full stomach is not good for digestion.

Do not do isometric stretches in the morning if you plan to work out on strength or flexibility later in the day. Isometric stretches may be too exhausting for your muscles if you do them twice a day. You must allow a sufficient time for recovery between exercises.

The whole early morning routine can take about 30 minutes for beginners and only a few minutes for advanced—after reaching the desired level of flexibility, you will need less work to maintain it. You should not get tired during the morning stretching. The purpose of this stretching is to reset the nervous regulation of the length of your muscles for the rest of the day. Remember: Do not work too hard because fatigue reduces your range of motion in dynamic movements, and if you overdo it, you will defeat the purpose of this exercise.

Usually, no special cool-down is needed after the early morning stretching. If, in doing a great number of repetitions, you manage to considerably raise your temperature and pulse rate, slow down the pace of the last sets and then spend a minute or two walking. If you have lots of time in the morning, you can also do some relaxed static stretches at the end of your morning stretch.

Stretching in your workout

In your training, use dynamic stretches right after waking up as your morning stretch, and later, at the beginning of your workout, as a part of a warm-up (Wazny 1981b). Do static stretches after dynamic exercises such as running, jumping, throwing, kicking, or wrestling that make up the main part of your workout, preferably in a cool-down. If you need to display static flexibility in the course of your workout or event, then do these exercises at the end of the warm-up.

A properly designed workout plan includes the following parts.

1. The general warm-up, including cardiovascular warm-up and general, dynamic stretching (no static stretches unless you are a gymnast and the routine you practice includes static flexibility displays, such as splits and bridges)

2. The specific warm-up, in which movements resemble more closely the actual subject of the workout

3. The main part of the workout, in which you realize your task for this workout

4. The cool-down

The whole warm-up should take no more than 30 minutes. Dedicate about 10 minutes of this time to dynamic stretching. Warming up should involve a gradual increase in the intensity of your exercises. Toward the end of a warm-up, use movements that resemble more closely the techniques of your sport or the task assigned for this workout.

In New York City I have seen people sitting on heaters in order to warm up before a kickboxing workout. Apparently they did not realize that warming up has to prepare all systems of the body in order for you to perform at top efficiency. It has to affect the heart, blood vessels, nervous system, muscles and tendons, and the joints and ligaments—certainly not just one area of the body! One of the best books on physical therapy (Hertling and Kessler 1996) has it right: "*Warm-up* is an increase in body heat by active muscle use for the purposes of lowering soft-tissue viscosity and enhancing body chemical and metabolic functions, to protect and prepare the body for more aggressive physical activity. . . . Active muscle [warm-up] is likely to be more productive than passive means of heating, because passive heating does not [adequately] enhance the metabolic and cardiac factors, which are also important."

Begin your warm-up with limbering up, such as joint rotations, starting either from your toes or your fingers. Make slow circular movements until the joint moves smoothly, then move to the next one. If you start from your fingers, move on to your wrists, followed by your elbows, shoulders and neck. Continue with twisting and bending of your trunk followed by movements in the hips, the knees, the ankles, and finally, the toes. If you start from your toes, the order is reversed. The principles are: from distant joints to proximal (to the center of the body); from one end of the body to the other (top to bottom or vice versa), ending with the part of the body that will be stressed most in the next exercise. This last principle applies to all parts of a workout.

Next engage in five minutes of aerobic activity such as marching or jogging combined with trunk twists, leans, arm swings, skips, knee raises, or shadowboxing—anything having a similar effect on the cardiovascular system. Flexibility improves with an increased blood flow in the muscles (Wazny 1981b).

Follow this with dynamic stretches—leg raises to the front, sides and back, and arm swings, for example. Do leg raises in sets of ten to twelve repetitions per leg. Do arm swings in sets of five to eight repetitions. Do as many sets as it takes to reach your maximum range of motion in any given direction. The total number of repetitions needed for reaching the maximal range of motion increases with age. It may take 15–25 repetitions for 8-year-olds to reach the maximum range in shoulder and hip joints but 30–45 repetitions for 17-year-olds (Raczek 1991). For properly conditioned athletes, even those who are much older, usually one set in each direction is enough warm-up, however.

Doing static stretches in the warm-up for a workout that consists of dynamic actions is counterproductive, and it certainly does not prevent injuries (Shrier 1999; Pope et al. 2000). The goals of the warm-up are: an increased awareness, improved coordination, improved elasticity and contractibility of muscles, and a greater efficiency of the respiratory and cardiovascular systems. Static stretches, isometric or relaxed, just do not fit in here. Isometric tensions will only make you tired and decrease your coordination. Passive, relaxed stretches, on the other hand, have a calming effect and can even make you sleepy. A proper warm-up improves the mechanical, chemical, and neural aspects of your muscles' function and thus prevents injuries, but an improper warm-up, including wrong stretching, may predispose you to injuries (Safran et al. 1989).

Some reasons not to do static stretches before exercise according to Shrier (1999; 2000):

—There is no scientific evidence that static stretching before exercise reduces the risk of injury.

—Even mild static stretching can damage muscle cells.

—Static stretching increases pain tolerance.

In the words of Dr. Shrier (2000), "It does not seem prudent to increase one's tolerance to pain, possibly create some damage at the cytoskeletal level, and then exercise this damaged anesthetized muscle."

For a period from several seconds up to five minutes following a static stretch you cannot display your top agility or maximal speed because your muscles are less responsive to stimulation—your coordination is off. Relaxed static stretches decrease strength by impairing activation of the stretched muscles for up to five minutes after the stretch and contractile force for up to one hour (Fowles et al. 2000). Relaxed static stretches impair the activity of tendon reflexes—several 30-second static stretches of the calf muscles reduce the peak force, the force rise rate, and the half relaxation rate of the Achilles tendon reflex (Rosenbaum and Hennig 1995).

Maximal force production is impaired for several minutes after strenuous stretching, whether static or ballistic bouncing. (Stretching is strenuous when you do it at the pain threshold and it is light when you feel a sensation of stretch, but not pain.) Kokkonen et al. (1998), showed that maximal force in knee flexion declined on the average by 7.3% and in knee extension by 8.1% after six 15-second static stretches even though 10–25 minutes passed between static stretching and strength tests. Maximal force of the legs may decline less or not at all if an athlete walks for a few minutes following static stretching and prior to resistance exercise, an inadvertent revelation due to poor design of a study by Morgan (2000). Reduction of activation, or imbalance in activity, that follows static stretching is more likely to cause an injury than a reduction in strength (Murphy 1991). (This applies to a single workout and not to long-term training. A long-term [3–12 weeks] stretching program may improve strength performance [Kokkonen and Lauritzen 1995; Wilson et al. 1992; Worrell et al. 1994].)

All of the above notwithstanding, East European sports training authorities consider alternating stretches with sets of resistance exercises (for either maximal strength or for muscular endurance) a very effective means for developing both flexibility and strength (Platonov 1997; Platonov and Fesenko 1990). You have to keep in mind that a) exercises developing maximal strength need not involve overcoming maximal resistance nor moving at a high velocity, and b) an athlete who wants to alternate resistance exercises with stretches needs to be well attuned to the effects of either of these exercises on his or her muscles. In such alternating work each set of stretches causes an increase of the range of motion over the initial value and each following set of resistance exercises causes a reduction in the range of motion, but the increases are larger than reductions so the final range of motion is considerably greater than the initial range (Platonov 1997).

Static stretching reduced drop jump performance and tended to decrease explosive force production. Proprioceptive Neuromuscular Facilitation (PNF) stretching has a similar effect but not statistically significant—mean drop jump performance reduced by 3.2% and mean explosive force production reduced 3.3% (Young and Elliott 2001). In Young and Elliott's study, just as in Morgan's, the tested athletes also walked for a few minutes between stretches and jumps, which may be the reason for such small decreases in performance.

> Caution: If you try to make a fast, dynamic movement immediately after a strenuous stretch, whether static or bouncing, you may injure the stretched muscles.

After the general warm-up you can move on to a sport- or task-specific warm-up. The choice of exercises in the specific warm-up depends on your sport and on the subject of the workout—different if developing strength is the subject, different if developing endurance, and different yet if learning a technique, with each technique requiring different warm-up and lead-up exercises. (Structuring workouts for developing those and other abilities and skills is explained in *Science of Sports Training: How to Plan and Control Training for Peak Performance.*)

A specific warm-up should blend with the main part of your workout. When the main part is over, it is then time for the cool-down and final stretching. Usually you would only use static stretches here. You can start with the more difficult static active stretches that require a relative "freshness." After you have achieved your current maximum reach in these stretches, move on to either isometric or relaxed static stretches, or both, following the isometric stretches with relaxed stretches.

Caution: Pick only one isometric stretch per muscle group and repeat it two to five times, using as many tensions per repetition as it takes to reach the limit of mobility that you have at this stage of your training.

After all the isometric stretches, you can do relaxed stretches for the same muscle groups—if you feel like it. The relaxed or static passive stretches permit staying in maximally extended positions longer than the isometric stretches. Doing relaxed static stretches after isometric stretches may increase your passive range of motion and reduce tension in static stretches further than using either type of stretches alone. After the final stretches, march or walk around the gym or track for a few minutes to help the neural regulation of your muscles return to normal.

This is the end of your workout. If you do not participate in any sports training, but still want to stretch, just skip the specific warm-up and the main part of workout. Do only the stretches, starting with the dynamic and ending with the static.

Question: I am 29 years old, I do the strength workout twice a week and I use the following exercises:

- warm-up: 5 minutes

- dynamic stretches

- squat (3 x 12)

- isometric stretch

- adductor flies (100 reps)

- good morning lift (3 x 12)

- relaxed static stretch

I pick only one exercise per muscle group both in isometric and static and I do it 3–5 times tensing in each time 3–5 times for three to five seconds. Is this sequence and method correct?

Answer: Yes, this is an example of a good sequence of exercises.

If you follow my advice to the letter, and the rest of your athletic training is run rationally, you should be able to display your current level of flexibility within a month without any warm-up. By *current level of flexibility*, I mean the level you normally display during a workout when you are sufficiently warmed up. Of course, it is still better to warm up before any exercises. Being able to do splits and high kicks without a warm-up does not mean that you are ready to exercise. Warming up lets you perform efficiently during your workout or sports event and speeds up the recovery afterward. Muscles prepared for work do not get as much mechanical and chemical damage as the unprepared ones.

After you attain the required reach of motion, you may reduce the amount of work dedicated to maintaining this flexibility. Much less work is needed to maintain flexibility than to develop it. You will have to increase the amount of "maintenance" stretching as you age, however, to counter the regress of flexibility related to aging.

The use of partners in stretching

The practice of using partners in stretching is a waste of time, and it is dangerous. The helper is neither stretching nor resting. The danger of using a partner in stretching is obvious. The partner does not feel what you feel. He or she can easily stretch you a bit more than you would like. If you feel pain and let your partner know about it, by the time the partner reacts, it can be too late.

Children and flexibility training

Preschool children (ages 2 to 5) do not need to dedicate as much time to flexibility exercises as older children and adults, who may have to spend as much as 5–15 minutes per workout on flexibility. Their bodies are so pliable that in the course of natural play they will put their joints through the full range of motion (Drabik 1996).

From the age of 6 to 10, the mobility of shoulder and hip joints is reduced. To prevent this reduction of mobility, children in this age range must do dynamic stretches for shoulders (arm raises and arm rotations in all directions) and hips (leg raises in all directions). Flexibility of the spine reaches its natural maximum at ages 8–9 (Drabik 1996). Striving to increase the spine's range of motion beyond the natural maximum, as well as repetitive bending and twisting of the spine, may cause all sorts of problems—stress fractures to the growth plates of the vertebrae, spondylolysis, spondylolisthesis, and slipped discs—resulting in lifelong back problems (Micheli 1990). Some gymnasts pay for their spine's great flexibility by wearing body braces and spending the rest of their life in pain.

Avoid static stretches of all kinds (passive, active, isometric) in children's training because excitation dominates over inhibition in a child's nervous system. This means that it is hard for children to stay still, relax, and concentrate properly on feedback from their muscles for periods as long as static stretches require (Drabik 1996). Isometric stretches require concentration and body consciousness to properly interpret sensations coming from the stretched and strongly tensing muscles so as not to injure them. Isometric stretches that start from the standing position, leading to the side split put sideward force on the knees. This force can, with repeated application, stretch the ligaments and deform joint surfaces of the knees and thus cause loose and knocked knees (Alter 1996).

> Caution: Do not do ballistic, isometric, and strenuous relaxed stretches before the second stage of adolescence because children's muscles do not resist stretching as much as those of adults and these kinds of stretches cause their ligaments to be stretched (Raczek 1991). Ballistic stretches, in which you bounce to increase your maximum stretch, are risky (Ciullo and Zarins 1983) and mostly useless.

Static active stretches, especially lifting the leg and holding it high without any support, compress the spine and may increase lordosis because they bend and twist the spine while the hip flexor (iliopsoas) of that lifted thigh is pulling at the lumbar vertebrae. If you have to do such leg lifts, as might be the case in gymnastics, for example, you should immediately follow them with exercises and stretches that correct lordosis (pelvic tilts, forward bends).

Ages 10 to 13 (before the growth spurt) is when you intensify flexibility training because children, by gaining mass faster than height, get stronger and more active. Increased activity without an increased amount and intensity of stretches may reduce their flexibility (Drabik 1996).

During the growth spurt (13 to 15), height may increase nearly one inch in a month. Micheli (1990) states that muscles and tendons do not elongate as quickly as growing bones and the resulting loss of flexibility leads to overuse injuries. Specifically, Micheli says, an excessive lumbar lordosis, leading to back injuries, results from bones of the spine growing faster than its muscles, and that pain in the kneecap, and eventually destruction of its cartilage, is caused by doing too much knee-bending when the quadriceps is tightened by the rapid growth of thigh bones (Micheli 1990). A large study on more than 900 high school students, however, suggests that loss of flexibility is not caused by growth but only associated with it (Feldman et al. 1999). In any case, stretches should target these muscles that are overly tight, otherwise the child will develop bad posture or get injured (Micheli 1990). During this first stage of adolescence all bones, ligaments, and muscles are weakened and you should therefore avoid stressing the trunk by many repetitions of bends and twists.

In the second stage of adolescence, after the growth spurt (15 to 19), you can intensify flexibility training once again and do sport-specific stretches in quality and quantity similar to those for adults (Drabik 1996).

L. P. Matveev (Matveyev [Matveev] 1981) points out that the effectiveness of flexibility training is greatest during childhood and teenage years, and warns against exceeding the ranges of motion permitted by normal joint structure. "Excessive development of flexibility leads to irreversible deformation of joints and ligaments, distorts stance and adversely affects motor abilities," he says.

The elderly and flexibility training

Can you improve your flexibility if you are fifty or sixty years old? Why not? Eighty-year-old people can. How far you can improve in absolute terms, i.e., what range of motion you can achieve, depends on the initial level of your flexibility and strength.

Past maturity both flexibility and strength decline, partly due to aging and partly due to inactivity (Bassey et al. 1989; Gersten 1991; James and Parker 1989). Strength and flexibility training can decrease the age-related loss of strength and maintain or restore flexibility (American College of Sports Medicine Position Stand 1998; Buckwalter 1997). Strength training alone, without any stretching—with resistance permitting maximally 6–10 repetitions without straining, at a full range of motion—can increase flexibility of the elderly (Barbosa et al. 2002).

Even elderly men and women over seventy years old can increase their flexibility (Brown et al. 2000; Lazowski et al. 1999). With strength training the elderly, even in their 90s, can increase their strength and muscle mass—not as fast and as much as young people, but they can (Fiatarone et al. 1990; Lexell et al. 1995), and the responsiveness to strength training determines the effectiveness of isometric stretches—the most intense stretches—as long as the structure of the person's joints is not an obstacle.

Ultimately, whether an elderly person can increase his or her flexibility depends on the individual.

To see if the structure of joints (shape of bones and length of ligaments) permits reaching the extremes of normal range of motion, perform tests such as those on pages 108 and 110. To see if a given kind of stretches works for you—try them and see. For example, to see if isometric stretches are effective and safe, try them. If contracting a stretched muscle helps to increase the range of motion upon relaxing this muscle, then the isometric stretches are effective. If repeating these stretches every couple or every few days does not cause a persistent muscle soreness, or pain, or weakness—then most likely they are safe. Similar trials can be made with other kinds of stretches.

* * *

In the following chapters you will find a practical demonstration of principles discussed up until now. The exercises are shown in the sequence that you should use in a workout: from dynamic movements to static ones, gradually moving from a vertical to a horizontal position, each exercise evolving from a previous one. You will find more than the absolutely essential number of stretches for a particular group of muscles. This way, in planning a workout, you have many exercises to choose from and arrange in a methodically correct sequence that suits the subject of the workout. This does not mean that you should do all of them in any of your workouts— one of each type of stretch for a given group of muscles is usually enough. So, in a workout you would do one dynamic, one isometric, and one relaxed stretch for the hamstring, for example. Consider the facilities where you will work out and what kind of exercises will precede and follow each stretch. You do not want to sit in a puddle to stretch your hamstring, for example. You do not want to directly change position from standing to lying down (or vice versa) without stretching in the intermediate positions.

Most photographs in the following chapters show only the final positions of stretches. To start doing any of these stretches you do not have to lean your trunk, spread your legs, or twist your arms as far as these photographs show.

3. Dynamic Stretching

Dynamic flexibility, the ability to perform dynamic movements within a full range of motion in the joints, is best developed by dynamic stretching. This kind of flexibility depends on the ability to combine relaxing the extended muscles with contracting the moving muscles. Besides perfecting intermuscular coordination, dynamic stretching reduces passive resistance to movement throughout the range of motion (McNair and Stanley 1996; McNair et al. 2001).

Fatigue usually reduces dynamic flexibility, so do not do dynamic stretching when your muscles are tired, unless you want to develop a specific endurance and not flexibility. Dynamic stretching is most effective when you carry it out daily, two or more times a day (Ozolin 1971). Russian researcher L. P. Matveev (Matveyev [Matveev] 1981) cites one experiment: One group of athletes did two sessions of dynamic stretching every day for five days, with thirty repetitions per session. Results (increases in dynamic range of motion) for that group were twice as great as for the group that followed a regimen the same in every respect except with a day of rest following each working day.

According to Matveev eight to ten weeks is sufficient to achieve improvement resulting from acting on the muscles. Any further increase of flexibility is insignificant, and it depends on long-term changes of bones and ligaments. Such changes require, not intensive, but rather extensive training, i.e., regular loads over the course of many years (Matveyev [Matveev] 1981).

Dynamic stretches are performed in sets, gradually increasing the amplitude of movements in a set. The number of repetitions per set is 5–15. The number per session needed to reach the maximal range of motion in a joint depends on the mass of muscles moving it—the greater the mass, the more repetitions. A reduction of range is a sign to stop. A well-conditioned athlete can usually make a set

31

of 40 or more repetitions at maximal amplitude (Matveyev [Matveev] 1981).

Do dynamic stretches in your early morning stretch (see page 19, chapter 2) and as a part of the general warm-up in a workout. (Stretching in the morning is just as effective as at any other time—provided you warm-up well [Matveyev {Matveev} 1981; Wazny 1981b].) On days you do not work out you still should do dynamic stretches twice every day—once in the early morning stretch and once more later in the afternoon. The afternoon stretching session can include the same dynamic stretches as the morning stretch. If you work at night and sleep during the day, do two sessions of dynamic stretching too, one after you wake up and one more a few hours later.

Start your movements slowly, gradually increasing the range and the speed of movements. Do not "throw" your limbs, rather, "lead" or "lift" them, controlling the movement along the entire range. Then, after you have nearly reached your full range of motion, you can increase the velocity of the limb so the last few inches of its trajectory can be less controlled—but still, the stretch should not be sudden. Logan and McKinney (1970) apply the principle of *specific adaptation to imposed demands* in the case of flexibility. This principle means that eventually, either at the end of the first set of dynamic stretches or in other sets, you should stretch at a velocity not less than 75% of the maximal velocity used in your actual skill, a kick, for example.

As a rule, synchronize your breath with stretches so you breathe out with flexing your spine or compressing your rib cage and breathe in when extending your spine and expanding your rib cage. This is how it is done in dynamic exercises of yoga—Suryanamaskar (Grochmal 1986). For example, breathe out when bending your trunk forward so you end your exhalation at the greatest stretch, but when bending your trunk to the back, breathe in.

Dynamic stretches

Neck

Usually you use no special dynamic stretches for the neck. What you have done at the beginning of your warm-up (doing joint rotations) should be enough.

Arms

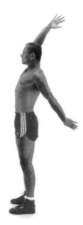

Swing your arms backward at varying angles.

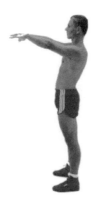 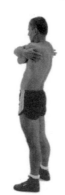 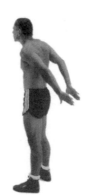

Crossing your arms in front, touch your shoulder blades with your hands, then straighten the arms and touch your hands behind your back. To increase the range of motion to the back, you can rotate your arms inward so the palms of your hands face out.

Legs

Beginners may have to start with a great number of repetitions—
four to five sets of ten to twelve repetitions per leg in any given direction, very slowly increasing the height at which the leg is raised.
You can switch the leg after each repetition or after a set. After a
month or two, you will notice that it takes less repetitions to reach
a maximum range of motion. Eventually one set of twelve repetitions in each direction, per leg, will be enough.

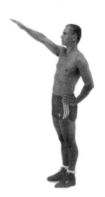 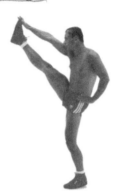

Leg raise to the front. With your hand as a target it is easy to evaluate your progress. Maintain good posture (straight trunk) and your
hand can serve as a stop for very dynamic (explosive) leg raises (see
pages 5 and 6). Start as low as feels comfortable. Keep your supporting leg straight, its heel on the ground if possible.

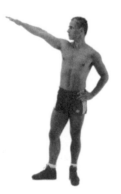 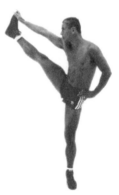

Leg raise to the side. The leg raise to the side is the same as a front
raise, except your arm is stretched to the side and you raise your leg
sideways.

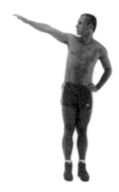 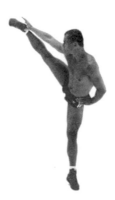

Another form of the side raise. This form is useful for martial art-ists. The foot of the leg about to be raised points forwards and con-tact with your palm is made by the side of the foot. Your hips will have a tendency to move to the back and your trunk will lean for-ward, which is all right, but do not lean forward any more than nec-essary. Gradually increase the height at which you place your hand, starting at hip level.

If the outside of your hips hurts when you do high leg raises to the side or side kicks, you need to tilt your pelvis forward while you kick. If you don't, you will jam the neck of your thigh bone into the cartilage collar at the upper edge of the hip socket. If you have *coxa vara* (a bending of the neck of the femur), you could also jam the greater trochanter against your hip bone.

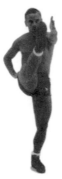

Leg swing from the outside to the inside. You can again use your hand as a target. Try to bring the leg as far as possible across your front.

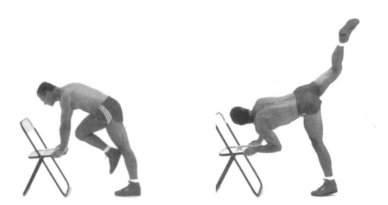

Leg raise to the back. Using any form of support at about your hip height, raise the leg as high as possible. Feel the stretching in front of your thigh.

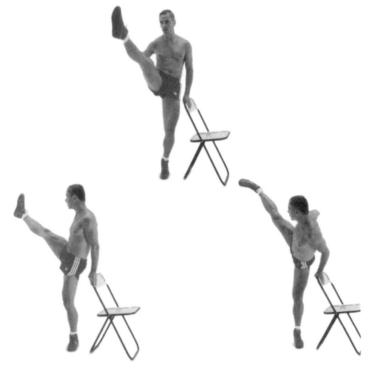

If using a support lets you raise your legs higher to the front and sides—use it.

Trunk

If your sports discipline requires a rapid twisting and bending (with great amplitude) of the trunk, add the following set of exercises to your stretching routines. You can expect to reach full mobility of the trunk (the joints of your vertebral column) in a given direction after 25–30 repetitions of a given exercise.

You can do dynamic stretches for the trunk standing or sitting. A sitting position is better because it isolates the joints of the trunk (vertebral column) from the leg joints. Also, rapid front and side bends in a standing position can become ballistic stretches and injure you.

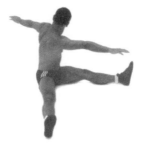

Rotations. Sit down and twist your trunk from side to side. Try to keep your hips and legs immobile.

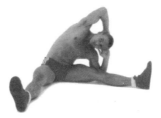

Side bends. While sitting down, lean from side to side.

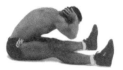

Forward bends. Lean forward from a sitting position. **Do not keep your back straight. Let it get round.** If you keep it straight, you will stretch your hamstrings instead of your back.

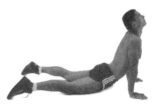

Bends to the back. Lie on your stomach and raise your trunk using your arms and the muscles of the back.

* * *

B. V. Sermeev (1968) studied dynamic stretches and recommends the following numbers of repetitions per set and per workout.

Arms: Maximal range of motion (ROM) is reached after 5–10 arm swings in any given direction, therefore these are minimum numbers per set; for developing dynamic flexibility the total numbers of repetitions recommended per workout are 30–40 for flexion-extension of the arm and 15–30 for arm circles; for maintaining flexibility 15–25 repetitions of full-range movements per workout are enough.

Legs and hips: Maximal ROM in any given direction of hip movements is reached after 10–15 leg raises in a given direction; for developing flexibility the total numbers of repetitions recommended per workout are 30–40 for flexion-extension of the thigh and the same for abduction of the thigh; for maintaining flexibility 15–25 repetitions of leg raises per workout are enough.

Trunk: Maximal ROM of the trunk (the joints of your vertebral column) in flexion and extension is reached after 25–30 repetitions of dynamic trunk stretches; for developing flexibility the total numbers of repetitions recommended are 40–70 per workout; for maintaining flexibility 30–40 repetitions per workout are enough.

4. Static Active Stretching

It is difficult to develop static active flexibility to the level of your dynamic or static passive flexibility. You have to learn how to relax stretched muscles and you have to build up the strength of the muscles opposing them, so that parts of your body can be held in extended positions. Although this kind of flexibility requires isometric tensions to display it, you should also use dynamic strength exercises for its development. In training to hold your leg extended to the side, for example, keep raising and lowering it slowly in one continuous motion. When you can do more than six repetitions, add resistance (ankle weights, pulleys, or rubber bands). After dynamic strength exercises, do a couple of static active stretches, holding the leg up for six seconds or longer, then do static passive flexibility exercises like isometric or relaxed stretches. Your static active flexibility depends on your static passive flexibility and static strength.

Caution: In the case of holding leg extensions, you must have a strong lower back. My rule of thumb for back strength is lifting comfortably—without psyching up and teeth grinding—at least twice your body weight in the deadlift. If you consider this excessive you are welcome to learn from your own experience.

If your sport requires only dynamic flexibility—for kicking, say—then you do not need static active stretches. Holding the leg up is not developing dynamic flexibility nor dynamic strength. It is developing a static active flexibility and static strength required of gymnasts but not something that kickers need.

Static active stretches that involve muscles of the back, such as leg extensions and trunk exercises, compress the spine, squeeze intervertebral discs, and may increase lordosis. This compression is especially harmful because it occurs when the spine is already bent, or bent and twisted. To minimize damage, do stretches such as forward bends and pelvic tilts immediately after these exercises. These stretches will relieve spasms of the back muscles and increase the amount of space between vertebrae.

Static active stretches and strength exercises

In the line drawings that follow (pages 41–48), you will see examples of strength exercises and static active stretches, each example followed by a photo of its result.

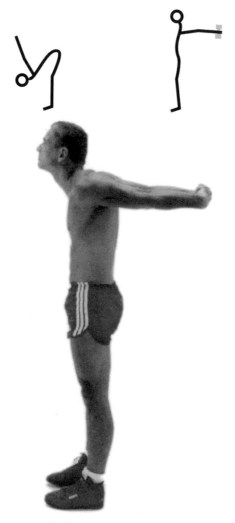

Arm extension to the back

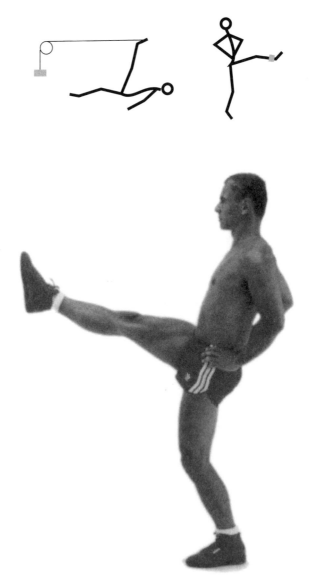

Leg extension to the front

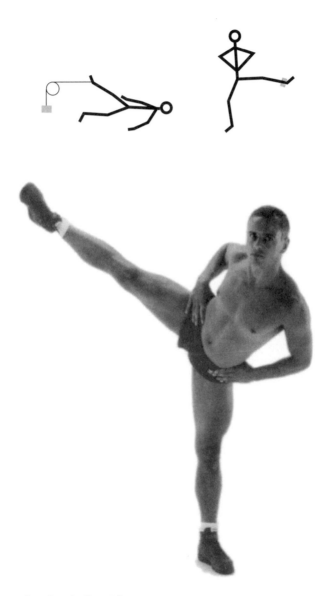

Leg extension to the side

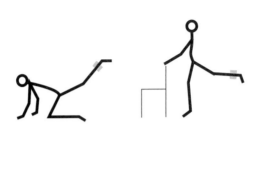

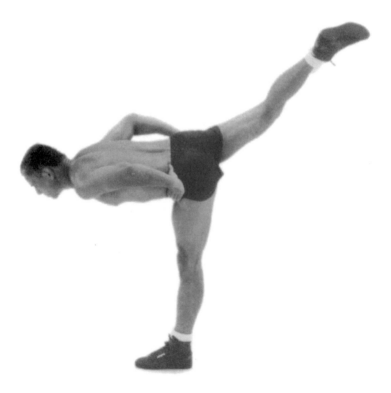

Leg extension to the back

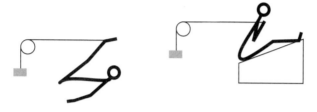

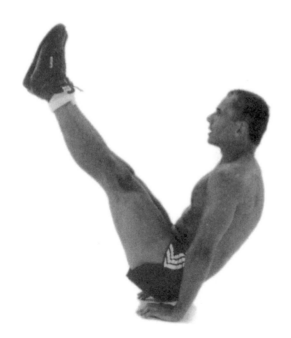

Hamstring and back stretch

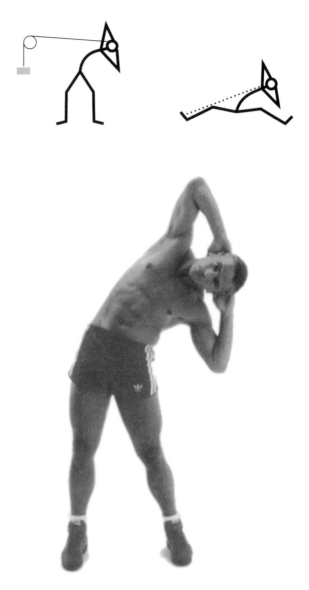

Side bend

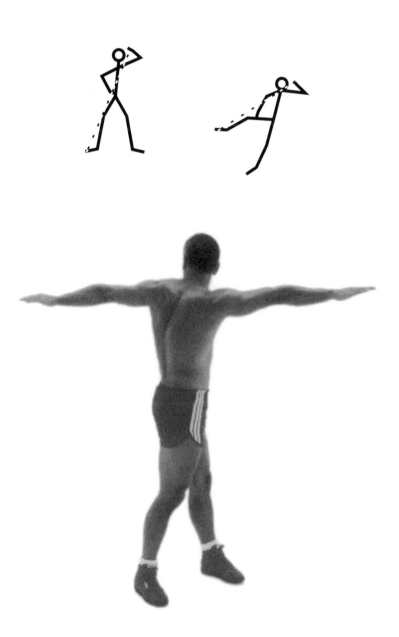

Trunk rotation

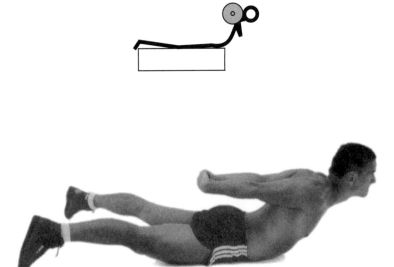

Back extension

5. Isometric Stretching

In this chapter and in chapter 6, "Relaxed Stretching," you will learn how to develop static passive flexibility. Passive flexibility usually exceeds active (static and dynamic) flexibility in the same joint. The greater this difference, the greater the reserve tensility, or flexibility reserve, and the possibility of increasing the amplitude of active movements. This difference diminishes in training as your active flexibility improves. Doing static stretching alone does not guarantee an increase of dynamic flexibility equal to the increase of static flexibility.

Static flexibility may increase when your muscles are somewhat fatigued. This is why you should do static stretching at the end of a workout.

Isometric stretching is the fastest method of developing static passive flexibility. It also improves active flexibility as well as strength in concentric, isometric, and eccentric actions (Handel et al. 1997). There are indications that it causes longitudinal growth of muscle fibers (Handel et al. 1997).

Isometric stretching is not recommended for children and adolescent athletes whose bones are still growing. Your bones should be mature and your muscles have to be healthy and strong for you to use isometric stretching.

> Caution: If you neglected your strength training, or were doing it incorrectly, isometric stretches may harm your muscles.

When you are not ready for isometrics

When a muscle is weak, due to improper strength training, or when it is stretched with too much force, it can become excessively damaged. Depending on the amount of stress and also on the strength of the muscle, this damage at a microscopic level can announce itself as muscle soreness, or it can amount to a complete muscle tear (muscle strain). To make the muscle stronger, you should do strength exercises with light resistance and a high number of repetitions. Do these exercises slowly. Make full stops at the beginning and at the end of each movement. You should do at least three sets, with a minimum of 30 repetitions per set, exercising the muscles that are most likely to be overstretched in your sport, or the ones that you intend to stretch isometrically in the near future. Good results are also brought about by doing long single sets of 100 to 200 repetitions.

You should do these high repetition exercises at the end of your strength workouts, after the regular heavy weights/low repetition exercises. After these high repetition exercises, you should do relaxed stretches for the same muscles.

Typically strength workouts or strength exercises for a given muscle group are done two or three times per week. How often you should do strength exercises depends on your reaction to them. If your muscles are sore the next day after every strength workout, even if you make some progress, it means that you exercise too often or too much. If you do not get muscle soreness but make poor progress, it may mean that you should exercise more often.

Be self-observant. Trial and error will teach you by what increments you can increase resistance and how frequently you can work out without getting sore. Muscle soreness is accompanied by loss of strength and by shortening of the muscles—most pronounced on the second day after the overly strenuous exercise (Clarkson et al. 1992). Those who exercise on a rigid schedule—for example, every other day—despite being sore after the previous workout may see their flexibility getting progressively worse rather than better.

It is difficult to state how long you need to perform the high repetition exercises after you have found out that your muscles are too weak for isometrics. To find out, you have to periodically test the reaction of your muscles to isometric stretches. If your muscles get sore, it means that they are still too weak.

When you are ready

Remember the caution in chapter 2, page 24: Pick only one isometric stretch per muscle group and repeat it two to five times, using as many tensions per repetition as it takes to reach the limit of mobility that you now have.

Russian researcher Matveev (Matveyev [Matveev] 1981) recommends doing isometric exercises four times a week, ten to fifteen minutes per day, using tensions lasting five to six seconds. The amount of tension should increase gradually and reach a maximum by the third and fourth second. In the particular case of isometric stretching you can hold the last tension, applied at your maximal stretch, much longer, for up to thirty seconds or sometimes even a few minutes. If you are just beginning isometric training, you should start with mild tensions, lasting two to three seconds. Increase the time and the intensity of tension as you progress. Any attempt to develop strength by isometric exercises only may lead to a stagnation of strength in only six to eight weeks. To develop exceptional strength as well as flexibility, combine isometric stretches with dynamic strength exercises such as lifting weights, using the same muscles. After a few weeks you may hit a plateau—regulating the tension and length of muscles will stop bringing any improvements in your stretches. Do not worry. Do your exercises concentrating on the strength gains you will achieve. These gains are shown by the increased time you can maintain a position, the amount of weight you can support, or the ability to stand up (slide up, walk up) from your attempts at splits. After some time, when your strength improves, you will notice a great increase in your flexibility.

If, as a result of isometric stretching, or any other exercises, your muscles hurt, reduce the intensity of the exercises or stop working out so you can heal completely. When the pain is gone, if isometrics as stretches or as strength exercises were the cause of the problem, prepare yourself for using them again by doing normal, dynamic strength exercises, gradually increasing resistance. If, for example, stretching your legs by isometric stretches caused pain in any of the leg muscles, stop exercising. Wait till the pain is gone, then try marching, running, running up an incline, climbing stairs, or doing squats. Later you can also do isolated strength exercises using the previously described method (see page 50) of low weight and a high number of repetitions. Do these exercises focusing on your weak or previously injured muscles. After these exercises and at the end of regular workouts, use relaxed stretches instead of isometric ones until you fully recover. Reintroduce isometrics into your training gradually, adjusting the number and the strength of the tensions, as well as the frequency, in the training week. Make adjustments according to what you feel in your muscles. When everything is all right, you will not feel any pain or soreness.

Several studies have been conducted to determine the number and frequency of the isometric tensions needed for the greatest strength gain, recalling that an increase of strength in isometric stretches means an increased length of muscles. In one study (Hettinger and Müller 1953), subjects with once-per-day sessions, using 66% of maximum contraction, had results equal to subjects using 80% of maximum contraction performed five times per day. Another study (Müller and Röhmert 1963) shows the greatest strength development when using five to ten maximal contractions per day, five days per week. Still other researchers (Fox 1979) report that using maximal contractions every other day is best. Russian researcher Matveev (Matveyev [Matveev] 1981) recommends doing isometrics four times a week, using maximal tension held for five to six seconds, and repeating each exercise three to five times. This is the method I followed because my body responded to it well. You may need a different number, strength, and weekly schedule of isometric tensions.

Isometric stretches, to increase flexibility, should be done at least twice a week, but it all depends on your recovery. If your muscles are sore then no isometric stretching should be done as long as soreness is felt. Wallin et al. (1985) recommends isometric or contract-relax stretching from three to five times a week for increasing flexibility, and for maintaining it only once per week.

Following is my weekly schedule, which suited me well at the time I posed for the photographs in this book. It may be less suitable for someone who works on endurance more often or does more or less resistance training than I did. This schedule serves primarily as an illustration of the overarching principle of training methodology, which can be summed up: "Work on speed or technique before working on strength, work on strength before working on endurance." Violating this principle leads to chronic fatigue, overtraining, or even injuries. Considerably fatigued muscles are less flexible than rested ones.

Monday—a technical workout dedicated to learning or practicing sports techniques, followed by light isometric stretching. Right after stretching, or later in the day, 20–30 minutes of aerobic running.

Tuesday—a strength workout consisting of strength exercises for the sport, followed by isometric stretching.

Wednesday—an endurance workout that develops endurance for the sport; no isometric stretching, although I might do relaxed stretches after the workout.

Thursday—day off

Friday—a technical workout followed by light isometric stretching. Right after stretching, or later in the day, 20–30 minutes of aerobic run.

Saturday—a speed-strength workout consisting of strength exercises with stress on speed of movements, followed by isometric stretching.

Sunday—day off

On Monday and Friday my stretching, as well as my whole workout, was lighter than on the following day (Tuesday, Saturday).

As you see in my schedule a technical or speed workout precedes a strength or endurance workout, a strength workout precedes an exhausting endurance workout, which is followed by a day of complete rest or active rest—some easy, fun activity.

A technical or speed workout should not be done on the day immediately following either an exhausting strength or an exhausting endurance workout, and a strength workout is not to be done after an exhausting endurance workout because such sequences of efforts lead to overtraining. *Science of Sports Training* gives the in-depth explanation of why the same exercises give different results depending on their sequence in a workout and in the weekly sequence of workouts.

If you lift weights, or do some other type of dynamic resistance training, do isometric stretches after your dynamic resistance exercises. On days when you work your legs, end your workout with one or two isometric stretches for your legs. On days when you work your upper body, do isometric stretches for arms and shoulders, for example.

If you "listen" to your body, you will be able to find the combination of exercises that works for you. For example, you may get best results doing isometric stretches every other day, or every third day. Any muscle soreness or pain is a signal to stop exercises. Do not resume your training if you feel any discomfort or even a trace of pain.

Isometric stretches

There are three methods of doing isometric stretches.

First method: Stretch the muscles (not maximally, though) and wait several seconds until the mechanism regulating their length and tension readjusts, then increase the stretch, wait again, and stretch again. When you cannot stretch any more this way, apply short strong tensions, followed by quick relaxations and immediate stretches (within the first second of relaxation) to bring about further increases in muscle length. The force of these tensions is from 50 to 100% of maximal voluntary contraction (Enoka et al. 1980). Hold the last tension for up to 30 seconds.

Second method: Stretch as much as you can, tense the stretched muscles and hold this stretched and tensed position until you get muscle spasms, then decrease the stretch, then increase it, tense it, and so on. The last tension should be held for up to five minutes. It makes some people scream.

Third method: This is the one I used to get the results shown in this book. Stretch the muscles, but not to the maximum, then tense for three to five seconds, then relax, and preferably within the first second and no later than the fifth second, stretch again. Alternatively, prior to stretching, maximally tense the muscles about to be stretched for a few seconds and then relax and within the first second stretch them. At the near maximal stretch, tense again for a few seconds to once again trigger the postcontractive stretch reflex depression and lower resistance to a stretch. Stretch further and further until you cannot increase the stretch.

> Tensing the muscles in a position in which they are neither maximally stretched nor maximally shortened—in which their tension can be greatest—is followed by a greater range of motion increase than tensing of already considerably stretched muscles.

Experiment to find out what strength and duration of the tension gives you the most stretch upon relaxation. For the greatest effect during a stretch tense the muscles opposing the stretched ones (Etnyre and Abraham 1986a). Some stretches—for example, standing stretches for the legs—cannot be done in this manner.

Gradually, in the course of several workouts, increase the time of the last tension to about 30 seconds. After a minute of rest, repeat the same stretch. Do three to five repetitions of a whole stretch per workout.

In all these methods, you should concentrate on the strength gains in a stretched position. When you cannot increase the stretch, concentrate on tensing harder or longer, or both. In time it will translate into a greater stretch. To increase the tension of a muscle at any given length—put more weight on it. In splits, not supporting yourself with your arms will help.

No matter which method of isometric stretching you choose, when doing the stretches, breathe naturally with deep and calm abdominal breaths. Inhale prior to tensing, exhale or hold the breath during maximal tension, inhale at the beginning of relaxation and, if convenient, exhale with further relaxation and stretch. (Of course, if you tense much longer than your normal exhalation, then you have to inhale and exhale several times during a tension.) In some positions it may not be convenient to exhale while relaxing and increasing the stretch between the tensions. In such cases inhale during relaxation and stretching. During the last stretch, if you end it with the phase of relaxation, try to exhale as you increase your range of motion.

How to select your stretches

Choosing the isometric stretches you should do depends on the form of the movements in which you need greater range of motion. Choosing which one to do first depends on the muscle group that you feel is the first obstacle. For example, you want to do a full front split and, as soon as you assume the initial position for the stretch, you feel the most stretch in the calf of the front leg. This signals that your first stretch should be for your calf. Another example: If you want to bring your outstretched arms behind your back while holding a stick in a narrow grip and the first resistance comes from elbow flexors—it means that the elbow flexors are the ones to stretch first.

* * *

Following are examples of isometric stretches for various parts of the body. Don't make the mistake of thinking you are supposed to do all these stretches. (See chapter 2, page 28.)

Neck

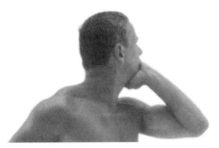

Turn your head to the side, block it with your hand, and try turning it back against the resistance of your arm. Relax and turn further in the same direction. Tense again. Hold the last tension for up to 30 seconds. Change sides.

A stretch for muscles[1] of the neck and the upper back: trapezius, sternocleidomastoideus, splenius capitis et cervicis, rectus capitis posterior major, semispinalis capitis et cervicis, obliquus capitis inferior, multifidus cervicis

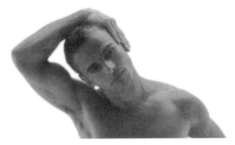

Lean your head toward the shoulder and block it with your arm. Tense the stretched muscles of the neck as if you are trying to straighten your head. Relax and bring it closer to the shoulder. Tense again. Hold the last tension for up to 30 seconds. Change sides.

A stretch for muscles of the neck and the upper back: sternocleidomastoideus, splenius capitis, scalenus anterior, scalenus medius, scalenus posterior, splenius cervicis, iliocostalis cervicis, longissimus capitis, levator scapulae

---

1   Listings of muscles throughout this chapter are based on anatomy manuals by S. Borowiec and A. Ronikier (1977) and by I. A. Kapandji (1974, 1982, 1987).

Forearm

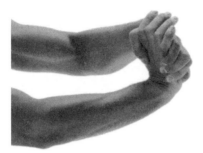

Bend your wrist. Hold your hand, tense, relax, flex more. Hold the last tension for up to 30 seconds. Change hands.

A stretch for the flexors of the hand: flexor carpi radialis, palmaris longus, flexor carpi ulnaris, flexor digitorum sublimis, flexor digitorum profundus

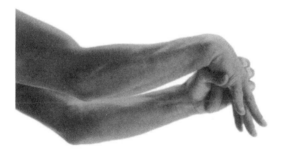

Bend your wrist in the opposite direction. Tense, relax, flex again. Hold the last tension for up to 30 seconds. Change hands.

A stretch for the extensors of the hand: extensor carpi radialis longus, extensor carpi radialis brevis, extensor digitorum communis, extensor carpi ulnaris

Arms, shoulders, chest

These stretches are for tennis players, swimmers, gymnasts, basketball players, team handball players, golfers, discus and javelin throwers, and hockey players. Students of certain martial arts (Indian muki boxing, wushu, sambo) that require a great mobility of the shoulders will find these exercises useful. Judo and sambo wrestlers, cyclists, skaters and hockey players can use stretches 2 and 4 as corrective exercises for a rounded back.

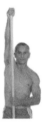

1. Hold the stick vertically in front of you. Tense the arm that holds the top end, as if to pull the stick down. Relax and, to stretch the raised arm, push the stick up with the arm that holds its bottom end. A stretch for the muscles of shoulder, chest, and upper back: teres major, teres minor, deltoideus, pectoralis major, pectoralis minor, rhomboideus, trapezius, latissimus dorsi

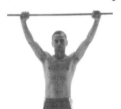
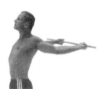

2. Starting from this position, bring the stick to the position behind your back and tense all the stretched muscles. Relax, bringing the stick to the front. Making your grip narrower, bring the stick to the back and tense again. When the grip is so narrow that you cannot lower your arms any more, stop and tense the stretched muscles for up to 30 seconds. This exercise stretches the front of the arms, shoulders and the chest: brachioradialis, biceps brachii, coracobrachialis, deltoideus, pectoralis major, pectoralis minor, teres major, serratus anterior, subscapularis.

> Caution: Do not force the stretch back beyond the point at which you can still tense the stretched muscles. Forced stretching can damage the shoulder joint capsule, which leads to shoulder instability and pain.

Outside rotation of your arms makes it easier to move them back or up. This is similar to rotating the thighs outside when spreading your legs. Rotating your arm externally makes the greater tuberosity of the humerus pass behind the acromion (a bone on top of the shoulder) instead of hitting it, so you can move the arm further back or up. Stretch both arms together so movements of your spine do not compensate for the range of movement in the shoulder girdle as they would in a single-arm stretch.

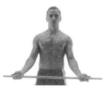 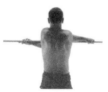

3. Change the grip. Twist the stick. Tense your upper back, shoulders and triceps. Relax. Move your hands further apart on the stick. Twist it again and tense the stretched muscles. Hold the last tension for up to 30 seconds. A stretch for the muscles of the upper back: trapezius, rhomboideus, latissimus dorsi

4. Through successive tensions and relaxations, crawl your hands toward each other. Hold the last tension for up to 30 seconds. Switch the position of your hands and repeat the exercise. A stretch for muscles of arms, shoulders, chest and upper back: triceps, anconeus, deltoideus, pectoralis major, latissimus dorsi, teres major, supraspinatus

The velocity of overarm pattern movements, such as baseball throws or volleyball serves and spikes, is related to the range of outward rotation of the arm (Sandstead 1968). The position of maximum outward rotation of the shoulder is where anterior shoulder injuries happen, however, so work on your shoulder flexibility with exercises that develop both flexibility and strength. Inward (internal) rotation of your arm with a bungee cord, or spring, or weight on a pulley, starting from a position of nearly maximal outward (external) rotation, will develop strength through the whole range of motion. Do this exercise with your arm bent at the elbow and keep your elbow close to your side. Hold the bungee cord or handle of the weight cable so its pull rotates your arm and moves your forearm away from your abdomen. Tense your muscles and bring your forearm to your abdomen.

If you let the bungee cord pull your arm to the limit of its outward rotation and tense from there, your tension can be used to override the stretch reflex (postcontractive stretch reflex depression) and so let you stretch the muscles that resist outward rotation of the shoulder. To stretch, first tense very hard in the position near the limit of the motion, then relax and within the first second of that relaxation let your arm be pulled or rotated further. Then you can repeat the cycle of tension and relaxation until you can't stretch any more. You can apply this type of stretching, which simultaneously strengthens muscles in the extreme range of motion, in other movements in the shoulder and in other joints.

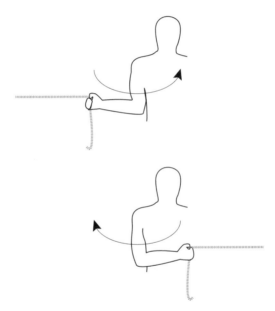

Inward (internal) rotation of the arm with a bungee cord starting from a position of nearly maximal outward (external) rotation (top drawing). This exercise should be balanced with outward (external) rotation of the arm (bottom drawing).

Legs

Stretches leading to the side split

If you have tried the test of flexibility potential (located on the last page of the book), you already know whether or not your joints will permit a side split. Here are some stretches leading to the side split. They are useful to martial artists, soccer players, skiers, hurdlers, dancers, skaters, gymnasts, and wrestlers (especially of jacket wrestling styles such as judo and sambo).

To do a side split from a standing position, flex your hips and knees in the same way and at least as much as when you are sitting on a low chair. This is similar to the so-called horse-riding stance. Your thighs should be parallel to the floor at any width, toes point forward, and chest up. At the beginning of a side split attempt, while you are standing in the horse-riding stance, your buttocks should be at the same level as your knees.

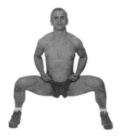 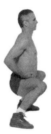

Inner thigh stretches. From this horse-riding stance, tense the inside of your thighs as if trying to "pinch" or squeeze the floor between your feet. Relax and spread your legs further. Keep repeating this cycle of tension and relaxation until you cannot lower yourself any more without pain. Hold the last tension for up to 30 seconds. When doing this exercise do not support yourself with your arms. Get out of the stretch without using your arms. This is a stretch for muscles of the inner thigh: adductor magnus, adductor brevis, adductor longus, gracilis, pectineus.

If you are a properly trained athlete you should not have any difficulty standing in a low horse-riding stance. After all, stances similar to it are encountered in many sports, for example, wrestling, weightlifting, volleyball, skiing, karate, basketball—just to name a few.

If you find this stance difficult, then gradually develop the flexibility and strength of your thighs, hips, and lower back in the horse-
riding stance. Start high and with feet only shoulder-width apart
and gradually progress lower and then wider. Keep your toes pointing straight ahead—if you let your toes point to the sides as you
widen the stance you will be grinding your knee cartilage (specifically the medial menisci). At all stages (heights, widths) you must be
able to do deep and calm abdominal breathing. If you rush and progress to wider and deeper stances before becoming comfortable at
the current stage, you may hurt your knees, subluxate or lock your
sacrum, and get lower back and neck pains. Bones of the pelvis—
the innominate bones, sacrum, and coccyx—move in relation to
each other in concert with phases of breathing (Walther 2000). (Yes,
they move, even though medical students are often taught that
there is no movement in the sacroiliac joint.) The muscles that stabilize the pelvis or cross the sacroiliac joint should not be kept
tensed hard in positions or at a time when that would interfere with
those movements.

You are ready to do an isometric side-split stretch when you can
stand comfortably at least a couple of minutes in a horse-riding
stance twice as wide as your shoulders with your thighs parallel to
the floor.

Question: When I attempt to do side splits, even though I believe I am using the correct posture, I feel a pain in the outer
part of my hip joints. Even though I feel that the muscles of my
inner thighs might stretch further, I feel severely limited by this
pain. It almost feels as though my joints are "locked," preventing any further movement. Is this condition normal?

Answer: Your complaint is typical for those who, while attempting the side split, do not flex their hip joints enough.
When your hips are not flexed enough they jam, and the only
way to spread your thighs wider is to tilt your pelvis forward
(the same way as when you lean your trunk so it is parallel to
the floor).

To do a side split from a standing position, the hip joint
should be flexed in the same way and at least as much as when
you are sitting on a low chair. This is similar to the so-called
horse-riding stance. The horse-riding stance averts irritation
of the upper brim of the hip socket and the resulting pain above
the hip joint.

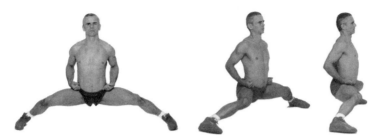

To get from this position to the full side split should take you about one month. At this stage people with weak knees may experience problems. In such cases, strength exercises for the muscles stabilizing the knees will help.

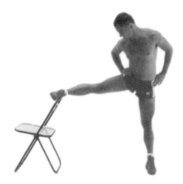

Another version of the inner thigh stretch. Gradually increase the height of the support or the distance from the supporting leg to the support. In the latter case, use something stable and not too high—for example, a pile of gymnastic pads—as your support.

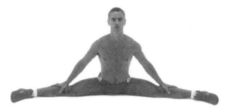

A full side split. Spend 30 seconds or more in this position tensing the inside of your thighs. Try lifting yourself off the floor by the sheer strength of your legs. Eventually you should be able to slide up from the split to a standing position without using your arms. Then you can try a full side split in suspension.

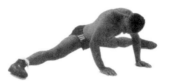

An exercise for a different kind of a side split—a side split with toes pointing upward. This is a stretch for the muscles of the inner thigh: adductor magnus, adductor brevis, adductor longus, gracilis, pectineus; and muscles of the buttocks: gluteus medius and gluteus minimus.

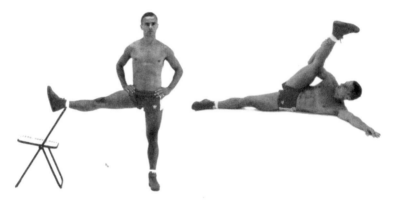

Two more versions of the previous stretch. Tense the muscles that feel stretched and relax them to increase the angle between your legs. Keep repeating this cycle of tension and relaxation until you cannot stretch any more without pain.

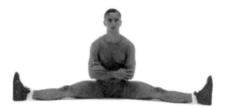

A side split with toes pointing upward

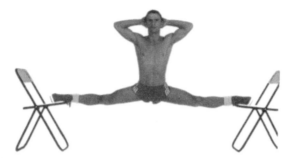

A full side split in suspension

Caution: A loss of balance may put your muscles out of commission for a year or more. Your first attempts should be done on objects low enough so that you can rest on the floor without tearing the muscles should you happen to lose your balance.

Side splits are not difficult. Anybody with normal range of motion in the joints of the hips and lower back can do them once learning the correct hip-pelvis alignment and with a little strength training of the adductors. Weakness of the adductors is the main obstacle to doing side splits. Weak adductors tense very strongly when you try to spread your legs in the straddle stance. The stronger they are the less tension, pain, and resistance there is while spreading your legs all the way to the floor. Generally the stronger the muscle the less activation it needs to support any given load (deVries 1980).

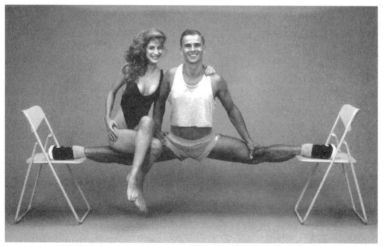

Another full side split in suspension

To balance stretches for the side split, which stressed the thigh adductors and internal rotators, do the following stretches for the muscles moving the thigh away from the body (thigh abductors) and muscles turning the thigh outward (external rotators of the thigh).

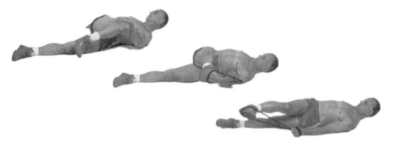

Outer thigh and hip stretches. Bring one leg across your center line. Tense the muscles of your outer thigh and hip as if you wanted to move your thigh up and out, then relax and bring the leg further across and down to feel more stretch. To feel the stretch mainly in the outer part of buttocks, bring the thigh up toward your chest. To stretch the front-outer hip (more stretch on the tensor fasciae latae), point the thigh down. These are stretches for muscles abducting the thigh: gluteus minimus, gluteus medius, gluteus maximus, tensor fasciae latae, piriformis.

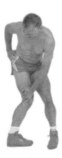

A stretch for muscles rotating the thigh outward. Bend your knee and turn your thigh and foot inward. Grab your thigh just above the knee and hold as you try to turn your thigh outward. Relax and turn your thigh (and your foot) more inward. This is a stretch for external rotators of the thigh (the muscles that limit its internal rotation): piriformis, obturatorius internus, obturatorius externus (only up to 40° of internal rotation of the thigh), quadratus femoris, pectineus (only up to 40° of internal rotation of the thigh), gluteus maximus, gluteus medius (posterior fibers), gluteus minimus (posterior fibers).

Stretches leading to the front split

If you have tried the test of flexibility potential (located on the last page of the book), you already know whether or not your joints will permit a front split. Here are some stretches leading to the front split. These stretches are important for cyclists, dancers, gymnasts, skaters, skiers, track and field athletes, wrestlers (especially judoka and sambo wrestlers), and martial artists.

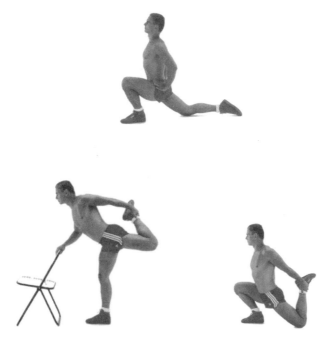

Front of the thigh stretches. Tense the muscles that bring your thigh forward and straighten your knee. Relax, stretch, tense again. Hold the last tension for up to 30 seconds. Change sides. These are stretches both for the muscles that bring the thigh up and forward (hip flexors), for example, in running, and for the muscles that straighten the knee: iliacus, psoas major, pectineus, obturatorius internus, adductor magnus, adductor longus, adductor brevis, gracilis, quadriceps (rectus femoris, vastus lateralis, vastus medialis, vastus intermedius), sartorius, gluteus minimus, tensor fasciae latae.

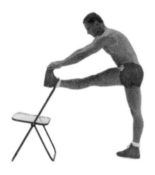
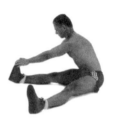

Calf stretches. Grab and pull your toes toward yourself. Point your foot forward against the resistance of your arms. Relax, pull the toes closer to yourself and start pointing the foot forward again. Hold the last tension for up to 30 seconds. Change legs. These are stretches for muscles of the calf: gastrocnemius, soleus, plantaris, flexor hallucis longus, tibialis posterior, flexor digitorum longus, peroneus longus, peroneus brevis. If you do these stretches with your knee bent, you stretch the soleus and with the knee straight you stretch both the soleus and gastrocnemius.

To strengthen and stretch muscles of the calf that limit the dorsiflexion of the ankle, as well as all muscles of your thighs and buttocks, do deep squats with feet kept flat on the ground. Do not bounce, just go down as low as possible and then raise up, tensing the stretched muscles. Do front and side lunges in the same fashion. If you cannot squat with your feet fully on the floor, it means that your soleus is too short. The remedy is to do increasingly deep squats or to do the calf stretches shown above.

Good forward range of motion in the ankle (dorsiflexion) permits you to lean more and reach with your arms further forward in a deep squat—like making a volleyball save or performing a wrestling leg pick.

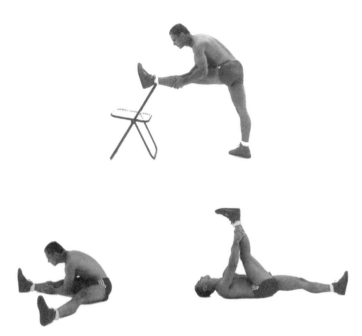

Hamstring stretches. Using one of the positions shown above, stretch your hamstring by decreasing the angle between your thigh and your trunk (in the sitting stretch) or increasing the angle between your thighs (in the standing and in lying stretches). Keep your spine straight to stretch your hamstrings and not your lower back and tilt your pelvis forward (push buttocks to the rear) to feel more stretch. Tense the hamstring as if to bring it back down, and then relax it. Pull your leg toward yourself, or if using a support, move the supporting leg further back. Tense again, relax and stretch more. Hold the last tension for up to 30 seconds. Change the leg. These are stretches for hamstrings, buttocks, and some of the pelvic muscles: biceps femoris, semimembranosus, semitendinosus, adductor magnus, gluteus maximus, gluteus medius (posterior fibers), gluteus minimus (posterior fibers), piriformis.

To increase the range of forward flexion in your hips and at the same time to strengthen muscles of the lower back, buttocks, and hamstrings do "good mornings" and stiff-leg deadlifts. Use weights light enough to let you move through the full range of motion.

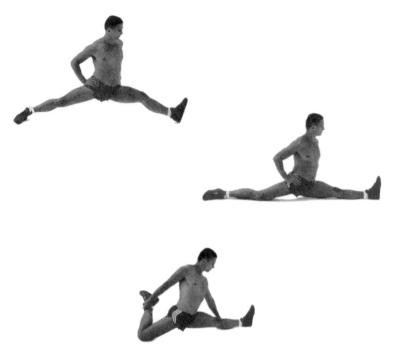

Pinch the floor, tensing the hamstring of your front leg, your quadriceps and the so-called runner's muscles of the rear leg. Relax and lower your hips. Tense again. Hold the last tension for up to 30 seconds. Change sides. These are stretches for muscles of the thighs, buttocks, and pelvis: iliacus, psoas major, quadriceps (rectus femoris, vastus lateralis, vastus medialis, vastus intermedius), sartorius, adductor magnus, adductor longus, adductor brevis, gracilis, pectineus, tensor fasciae latae, obturatorius internus, gluteus maximus, gluteus medius, gluteus minimus.

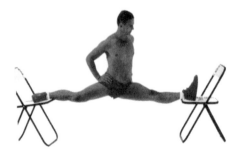

Full front split in suspension

Splits and high kicks

As a kicker, why should you be interested in doing a front split—a static stretch nonspecific for kicking that requires static flexibility while kicks require dynamic flexibility? Being able to do the front split facilitates (though it is not necessary for) learning high side and roundhouse kicks—the position of legs in a front split is the same as in high side and roundhouse kicks (the rear leg in this split corresponds to the kicking leg and the front leg to the supporting leg). If you can do the front split, you can practice the high side and high roundhouse kicks slowly enough to control and correct your body alignment, especially of the supporting leg in relation to the kicking leg and of the trunk in relation to the legs.

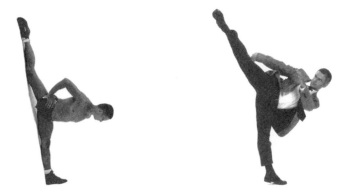

Front split (rotated) and a high roundhouse kick

The side split, if done according to my method of developing flexibility and strength both at the same time, strengthens the muscles of the inner thigh. These are the muscles of the supporting leg that are stressed when you do high kicks. During a kick the kicking leg displays only dynamic flexibility but the stretch on the supporting leg is more like a static stretch, albeit short, even abrupt. The inner thigh of the supporting leg tenses while being stretched by the momentum of your whole body moving toward a target. To strengthen the muscles of the inner thigh you can either tense them in a wide straddle stance and eventually in a side split or you can do resistance exercises such as adductor flyes and adductor pulldowns (shown on the video *Secrets of Stretching* available from Stadion Publishing).

Trunk

Following are stretches for track and field athletes (throwers), wrestlers, judoka, gymnasts, dancers, and tennis players.

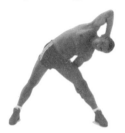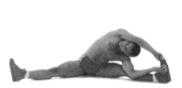

Side bends. Do not twist or lean forward. Move only to the side. Tense the stretched side as if to straighten up, relax and try leaning further to the side. Hold the last tension for up to 30 seconds. Change sides. These are stretches for muscles of the side of the abdomen and of the back: quadratus lumborum, longissimus dorsi, iliocostalis, obliquus abdominis externus, obliquus abdominis internus, psoas major.

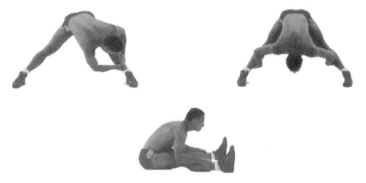

Lower back and hamstring stretches. Grab your legs and tense your back as if trying to straighten up. Relax, lean forward, and tense again. Hold the last tension for up to 30 seconds. To feel the stretch in the muscles of your back, round it slightly. Keeping your back straight stretches mostly your hamstrings.

These are stretches for the muscles of the back, buttocks, and hamstrings: longissimus dorsi, iliocostalis, multifidus, gluteus maximus, gluteus medius, adductor magnus, biceps femoris, semitendinosus, semimembranosus, piriformis, and muscles of the calves.

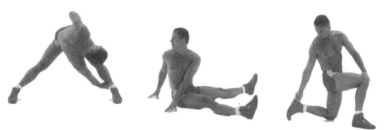

Trunk rotations. Twist (rotate) your trunk and grab your foot or put your hands on the ground. Tense the stretched muscles of your trunk, relax, and twist further. Tense again, relax, stretch and hold the last tension for up to 30 seconds. Change sides. These are stretches for muscles of the back and the abdomen: semispinalis, multifidus, transversospinalis, obliquus abdominis externus, obliquus abdominis internus.

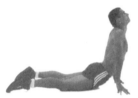

Abdomen stretch. Tense your abdomen as if trying to pull your hips forward and down. Relax, lower your hips, and tense again. Hold the last tension for up to 30 seconds. This is a stretch for the front of the abdomen, muscles on the front of the spine and the inside of the pelvis: rectus abdominis, obliquus abdominis externus, obliquus abdominis internus, quadratus lumborum, iliacus, psoas major, psoas minor.

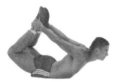

A more intense version of the previous stretch also affecting the front of the thighs. Usually your lower back will get very tense while you do these abdomen stretches. You can even get cramps. To relax the back, do the following "counterstretch," which you can do without tensing.

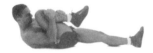

Recap

Isometric stretches are strenuous exercises requiring adequate rest between applications. For best results, supplement them with dynamic strength exercises as described in this chapter on page 50. In the workout, all dynamic exercises must precede the isometrics with few exceptions. (One example of an exception: You can include isometric tension involving multiple joints before speed-strength actions because such tensions can act as a stimulating factor [Gullich and Schmidtbleicher 1996; Siff and Verkhoshansky 1999]. If you elect to do this, the isometric tension has to be done in a position similar to that in which the maximal force is to be generated in the following speed-strength action.) You should do the isometric stretches after all the dynamic exercises rather than before because of the adverse effect on coordination that isometrics have.

Remember—a partner in stretching can cause an injury. If you need someone's help in doing any stretches, it means that you are not ready for them. It is better to go slowly but steadily.

6. Relaxed Stretching

Relaxed stretches are yet another means of developing static passive flexibility. Although much slower than isometric stretches, relaxed stretches have some advantages over isometrics. They do not cause fatigue and you can do them when you are tired. Problems are unlikely. There are two major drawbacks: your muscular strength in extended positions for all practical purposes does not increase as a result of relaxed stretching; and relaxed stretches are very slow. The same person who, in using isometrics, gets into a full side split in 30 seconds without a warm-up may take up to ten minutes of relaxed stretching (with no warm-up) to get to this same level. Within a couple of months of doing relaxed stretches this time gets shorter. After some more months it may take you from one to two minutes to do a full split. (With a good warm-up, of course, you can do it at once.)

In your workout, do relaxed stretches at the end of a cool-down just before the final walk or march. Do them after isometric stretches or instead of them. If you have enough time in a day, you can also do them whenever you feel like it, without a warm-up.

Relaxed stretches decrease strength by impairing activation of the stretched muscles for up to five minutes after the stretch and the contractile force for up to one hour (Fowles et al. 2000).

In doing these stretches, assume positions that let you relax all your muscles. This is the opposite of what you do in isometric stretches. Some isometric stretches are done in positions designed to maximally tense the stretched muscles—for example, by placing your weight on them as in side and front split stretches. In relaxed stretching you want as little weight on your muscles as possible. In splits, lean the body forward and support it with your arms. Relax completely. Think about slowly relaxing all your muscles. Do not think about anything energetic or unpleasant. Look in the direction of the stretch and breathe calmly, with deep abdominal breaths.

Usually it is easier to increase a stretch during exhalation—except when a stretch involves bending the spine backward. This is how it is done in yoga postures (Grochmal 1986). So, if you twist your back and neck, or just your neck, and raise your head to look up and behind yourself as far as you can, you will stretch and see further at inhalation. If during the same twist you look down (tip your head down), you will stretch and see further at exhalation.

Relaxing into a stretch, at some point you will feel resistance. Wait in that position patiently and after a while you will notice that you can slide into a new range of stretch. After reaching the greatest possible stretch (greatest at this stage of training), hold it; feel the mild tension in stretched muscles. Get out of the stretch after spending about 30 seconds in the final position. You can stay in the stretch longer—a minute or two—but for increasing the range of motion the most effective duration of relaxed stretches is 30 seconds (Bandy and Irion 1994), and the most effective frequency is once per day (Bandy et al. 1997). Do not stay in a stretch until you get muscle spasms. You can repeat the stretch after a minute.

* * *

Following are examples of relaxed stretches for various parts of the body. Don't make the mistake of thinking you are supposed to do all these stretches. (See chapter 2, page 28.)

Relaxed stretches

Most of the following relaxed stretches look similar to the isometric stretches for the same muscles. The difference is that in the relaxed stretches the stretched muscles are not tensed to override the stretch reflex. In relaxed stretches, you pull gently and continuously on the stretched (and relaxed) body part, unlike in isometric stretches in which you pull strongly against the alternately tensed and relaxed muscles.

Neck

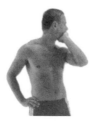

Put your hand on your cheek or your chin. Turn your head to the side. Gently pull with your hand to increase the range of motion.

Muscles[1] stretched: trapezius, sternocleidomastoideus, splenius capitis et cervicis, semispinalis capitis et cervicis, rectus capitis posterior major, obliquus capitis inferior, multifidus cervicis

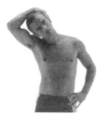

Put your hand on the side of your head. Lean your head toward the shoulder. Gently pull with your hand to increase the stretch.

Muscles stretched: sternocleidomastoideus, splenius capitis et cervicis, scalenus anterior, scalenus medius, scalenus posterior, iliocostalis cervicis, longissimus capitis, levator scapulae

---

[1]   Listings of muscles throughout this chapter are based on anatomy manuals by S. Borowiec and A. Ronikier (1977) and by I. A. Kapandji (1974, 1982, 1987).

Forearm

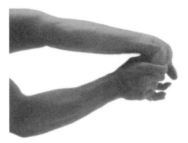

Bend your wrist, gently pulling with your other hand to increase the stretch.

A stretch for the flexors of the hand: flexor carpi radialis, palmaris longus, flexor carpi ulnaris, flexor digitorum sublimis, flexor digitorum profundus

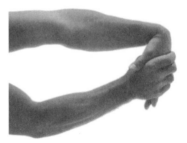

Bend your wrist in the opposite direction, gently pulling with your other hand to increase the stretch.

A stretch for the extensors of the hand: extensor carpi radialis longus, extensor carpi radialis brevis, extensor digitorum communis, extensor carpi ulnaris

Arms, shoulders, chest

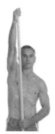

Hold the stick vertically in front of you. Relax the raised arm, and to stretch it, push the stick up with the arm that holds its bottom end.

A stretch for the muscles of shoulder, chest, and upper back: teres major, teres minor, deltoideus, pectoralis major, pectoralis minor, rhomboideus, trapezius, latissimus dorsi

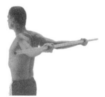

Bring the stick to the position behind your back, using the narrowest grip possible. Do not force the stretch beyond the sensation of a pleasant stretch.

Caution: Forced stretching can damage the shoulder joint capsule, which leads to shoulder instability and pain.

A stretch for muscles of the front of the arms, shoulders, and the chest: biceps brachii, brachioradialis, coracobrachialis, deltoideus, pectoralis major, serratus anterior, subscapularis

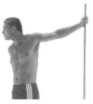

You can stretch the same muscles doing this stretch. Note the outside rotation of the arm, which makes it easier to move the arm back or up.

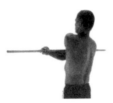

Change your grip on the stick and twist it.

A stretch for muscles of the upper back: trapezius, rhomboideus, latissimus dorsi

This is another form of the upper back stretch.

Crawl your hands on your back as far as you can.

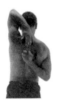

Grab your hands behind your back. If you cannot, use a piece of rope or a stick to crawl your hands toward each other. In turns, pull down the upper hand, then pull up the lower hand to feel a good stretch.

Muscles stretched: triceps, anconeus, deltoideus, pectoralis major, latissimus dorsi, teres major, supraspinatus

Remember that stretching both your arms together eliminates the influence of movement in the spine on the range of motion in your shoulder girdle.

Legs

Stretches leading to the side split

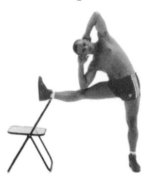

Place your leg on any support. Either lean toward this leg or move the other leg away from the support if this support is stable enough.

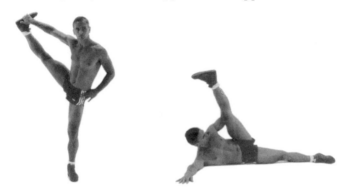

You can also lift your leg with your hand.

Stretches for muscles of the inner thigh: adductor magnus, adductor brevis, adductor longus, gracilis, pectineus

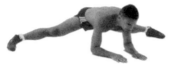 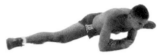

Stretch the muscles of both your inner thighs in this position. Shift your weight between your legs and arms to get the best stretch. When your legs tense, help them relax by putting most of your weight on your arms. When the legs relax, slide into a greater stretch by shifting your weight back.

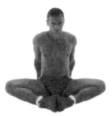

Here is one more, even milder inner thigh stretch. Sit down, bend your knees and pull your feet together. Now, lower the thighs using only the strength of the muscles that abduct and rotate them externally. Do not push with your hands.

Stretches for muscles of the inner thigh: adductor magnus, adductor brevis, adductor longus, gracilis, pectineus

To balance stretches for the side split (stretches for the thigh adductors and internal rotators), do the following stretches for the thigh abductors and the external rotators of the thigh.

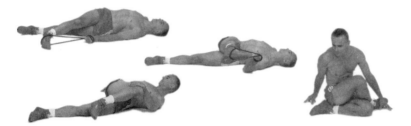

Outer thigh and hip stretches. Bring one leg across your center line to feel a stretch in your outer thigh and hip. To stretch the front-outer hip (more stretch on the tensor fasciae latae), point the thigh down. To feel the stretch mainly in the outer part of buttocks, bring the thigh up toward your chest. A stretch for muscles abducting the thigh: gluteus minimus, gluteus medius, gluteus maximus, tensor fasciae latae, piriformis

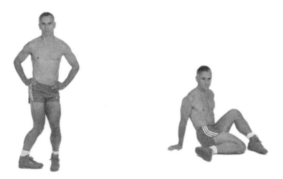

Stretches for muscles rotating the thigh outward. Standing upright bend your knee and turn your thigh and foot inward. Alternatively, you can stretch the same muscles while sitting with legs bent at the knees and feet about shoulder width apart. Lean back a little and support your trunk with your arms by placing your hands on the floor behind your hips. Attempt to touch the floor between your legs with the knee. These are stretches for external rotators of the thigh (the muscles that limit its internal rotation): piriformis, obturatorius internus, obturatorius externus (only up to 40° of internal rotation of the thigh), quadratus femoris, pectineus (only up to 40° of internal rotation of the thigh), gluteus maximus, gluteus medius (posterior fibers), gluteus minimus (posterior fibers).

Stretches leading to the front split

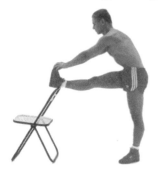 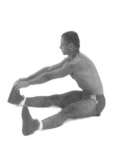

Calf stretches. Pull your toes toward yourself. Feel the stretching in the muscles of the calf: gastrocnemius, soleus, plantaris, flexor hallucis longus, tibialis posterior, flexor digitorum longus, peroneus longus, peroneus brevis.

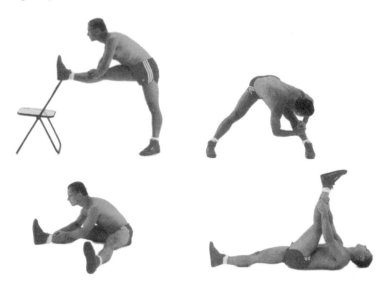

Hamstring stretches. Using any of the above shown positions, stretch your hamstrings. Keep your back straight to make sure you stretch mainly the hamstrings. Tilt your pelvis forward (push buttocks to the rear) to feel more stretch.

Muscles stretched: biceps femoris, semimembranosus, semitendinosus, adductor magnus, gluteus maximus, gluteus medius, piriformis

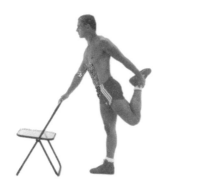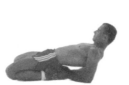

Front of the thigh stretches. These are stretches for the muscles of the front of the thigh and the so-called runner's muscles (hip flexors) originating inside the pelvis and in front of the spine: iliacus, psoas major, rectus femoris, quadriceps (vastus lateralis, vastus medialis, vastus intermedius), sartorius, adductor magnus, adductor longus, adductor brevis, gracilis, pectineus, tensor fasciae latae, obturatorius internus, gluteus minimus.

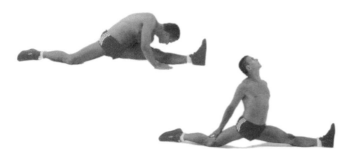

Sit in the front split. Lean your trunk forward and backward to stretch all the muscles of the thigh, buttocks, and pelvis.

Muscles stretched: iliacus, psoas major, rectus femoris, vastus lateralis, vastus medialis, vastus intermedius, sartorius, adductor magnus, adductor longus, adductor brevis, gracilis, pectineus, tensor fasciae latae, obturatorius internus, gluteus maximus, gluteus medius, gluteus minimus, biceps femoris, semimembranosus, semitendinosus, piriformis

Trunk

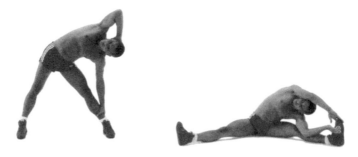

Side bends. Bend your trunk to the side. Do not twist or lean your trunk forward.

These are stretches for the muscles of the back and the side of the abdomen: quadratus lumborum, longissimus dorsi, iliocostalis, obliquus abdominis internus, obliquus abdominis externus, psoas major.

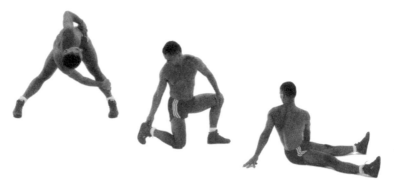

Trunk rotations. Rotate your trunk as far as it takes to feel a mild stretch. You can increase the stretch and help yourself keep it by putting your hand on your leg or on the floor.

Muscles stretched: obliquus abdominis externus, obliquus abdominis internus, semispinalis, multifidus, transversospinalis

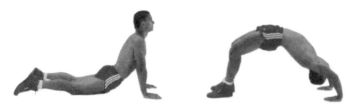

Abdomen stretches. These stretches are for the front of your abdomen and the muscles on the front of the spine and the inside of the pelvis: rectus abdominis, obliquus abdominis externus, obliquus abdominis internus, quadratus lumborum, iliacus, psoas major, psoas minor.

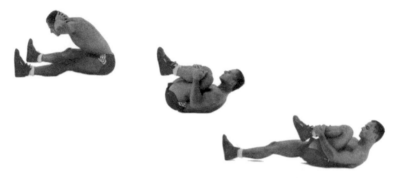

Lower back stretches. Stretch as much as it takes to relax the muscles of the back and not stretch its ligaments. Stretching the ligaments of the back weakens it. This is why you will not see here a relaxed stretch for the back in a standing position. The weight of the upper body hanging on your rounded and relaxed spine can stretch its ligaments. In the sitting stretch, to feel stretching in the muscles of your back, round it slightly. In the sitting stretch, keeping your back straight stretches mostly your hamstring.

Muscles stretched: longissimus dorsi, iliocostalis, multifidus

7. Sample Workout Plans

Here you get examples of how to choose exercises depending on the task of your workout and when to do them in the course of the workout. You will find several sport disciplines listed. Each is represented by one workout with the task common for that discipline.

These are just examples and not prescriptions. In a professionally run training process, no workout is the same. Each workout has either a different task or the task is realized by a different means every time. Different tasks and different means of their realization are assigned to workouts depending on the age, class, and condition of the athletes. In planning a workout the coach has to take into consideration the workouts done thus far, the next tasks that need to be done, when the athletes need their form to peak, and much more. To put it simply: your skill level and condition change from workout to workout, and so do your exercise needs.

The proper sequence of stretches in a workout is: dynamic, static active, isometric, relaxed. You do not have to do all these types of stretches in a workout. You can skip the ones that you do not need but do not alter the order unless you have a good reason and know what you are doing. For example, it sometimes may make sense to do a static stretch before dynamic stretch (but not before some high power or maximal force movements, such as powerful kicks).

In the following examples you will see only the flexibility exercises related to the task of the workout. The exercises of the main part of the workout are not shown.

Discipline: Track and Field—Hurdles. Task of the workout: The technique of passing the hurdles; no work on the start from the blocks or on the finish

General warm-up

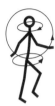 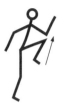 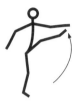

Jogging with rota-   March with knee   March with leg   March with leg
tions of the joints   raises   raises to the front   raises to the side

Specific warm-up

 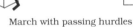

March with passing hurdles

Main part

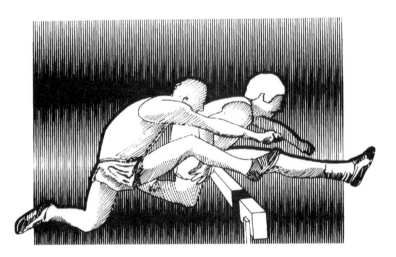

Cool-down

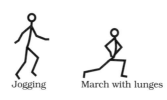

Jogging   March with lunges

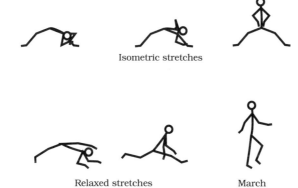

Isometric stretches

Relaxed stretches   March

Discipline: Gymnastics. Task of the workout: The development of flexibility and the perfection of the handstand (a task usually realized with children nine to ten years old)

General warm-up

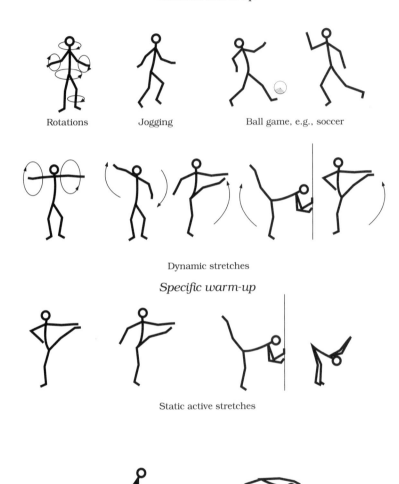

Rotations   Jogging   Ball game, e.g., soccer

Dynamic stretches

Specific warm-up

Static active stretches

Relaxed stretches

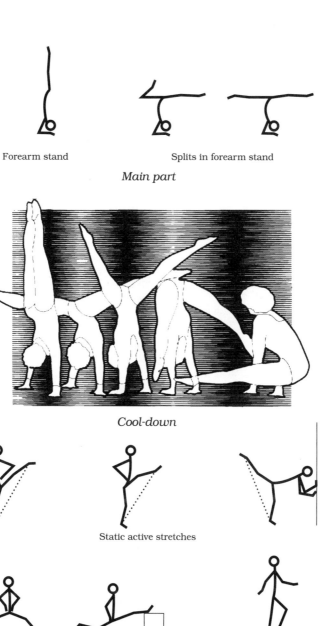

Forearm stand   Splits in forearm stand

Main part

Cool-down

Static active stretches

Isometric stretches   March

Discipline: Kickboxing. Task of the workout: The high round-house kick

General warm-up

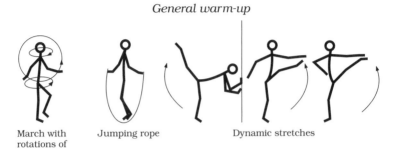

March with   Jumping rope   Dynamic stretches
rotations of
the joints

Specific warm-up

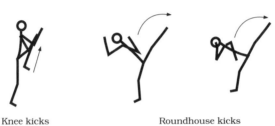

Knee kicks   Roundhouse kicks

Main part

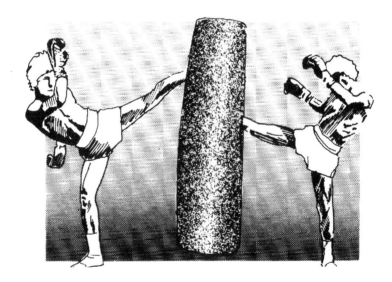

Cool-down

Front lunges   Side lunges   Isometric stretches

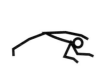

Relaxed stretches   Jumping rope

Discipline: Judo. Task of the workout: Teaching O-Soto-Gari (big outside sweep)

General warm-up

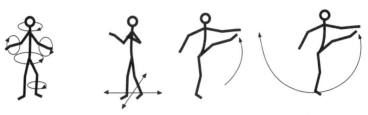

Rotations of   Judo steps   Dynamic stretches
the joints

Specific warm-up and main part of the workout

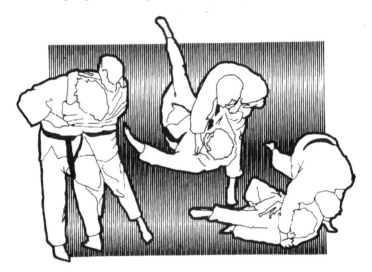

Cool-down

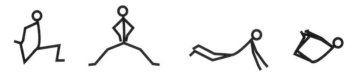

Isometric stretches

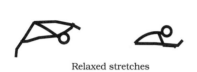
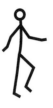

Relaxed stretches   March

Discipline: Bodybuilding. Task of the workout: Developing strength in the upper back, chest, forearms and lower legs

General warm-up

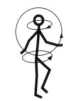 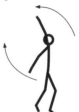

March with rotations of the joints   Dynamic stretches

Specific warm-up and main part of the workout

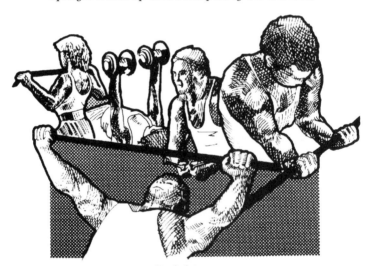

Cool-down

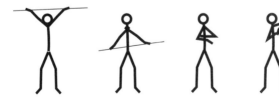

Isometric stretches

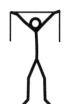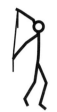

Relaxed stretches

Discipline: Swimming. Task of the workout: Speed in the butterfly stroke

General warm-up

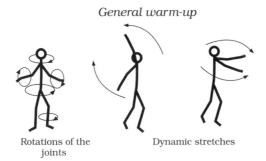

Rotations of the   Dynamic stretches
joints

Specific warm-up, main part and most of the cool-down in the pool

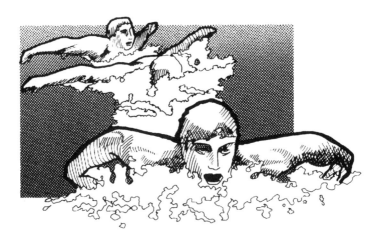

Cool-down

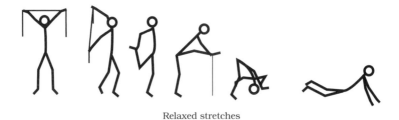

Relaxed stretches

8. All the Whys of Stretching

In this chapter, you will learn the whys of flexibility and stretching. This method of developing flexibility works for you regardless of whether or not you understand its physiological basis, as long as you do the exercises exactly as prescribed in chapters 1–6. Nevertheless, the more you know, the better your choice of exercises and the greater the likelihood of getting the results you want. Information—good information!—also gives you the basis for countering bad advice you may receive. Note this well: Mental rigidity—the inability to abandon fixed ideas while solving problems, a sign of low intelligence—is usually accompanied by a low level of physical flexibility—perhaps due to the connection between flexibility and coordination (Matveyev [Matveev] 1981). Coordination is considered a motor expression of intellect (Wazny 1981a).

Flexibility is the ability to perform movements of any amplitude (extent, or range) in a joint or a group of joints. Greater range means greater flexibility.

A high level of overall flexibility helps one to perform economically in fencing, and in various types of wrestling—Greco-Roman, freestyle, judo, sambo, shuai-chiao.

Certain sports—e.g., gymnastics, javelin throw, kickboxing—require a maximal development of flexibility in all or some of the major joints just for the execution of their basic techniques. Just the reverse is true in some others. The greater the flexibility of some joints, the worse performance. For example, long-distance runners lose running economy with greater dorsiflexion of the foot and external rotation in the hip joint (Craib et al. 1996).

In sports calling for a generation of maximum power in movement, before punching, jumping, throwing or hitting a ball, or putting the shot athletes instinctively make a movement in the opposite direction, knowing that a prestretch will increase their power. This is called stretch-shorten cycle. In dynamic concentric actions muscles work best if you contract them from an optimal stretch. Longer or more extended muscles can exert force on the object (ball, shot, fist) on a longer path and thus for a longer time, accelerating it more.

Poor flexibility of some muscles may contribute to injuries in some activities or sports. For example, in a study by Witvrouw et al. (2001) athletes with patellar tendinitis (jumper's knee) tended to have lower flexibility of their quadriceps (range of motion 86.0° [standard deviation 12.4°]) than athletes without patellar tendinitis (132.6° [standard deviation 14.9°]). In the case of rowing, hamstrings too short to permit as much anterior rotation of the pelvis as it takes to keep the lumbar spine from flexing more than 50% of its maximum range of flexion at the catch phase of the rowing stroke contribute to hypermobility of the lumbar spine (Reid and McNair 2000). Hypermobility of the lumbar spine correlates strongly with low back pain in rowers (Howell 1984). Increasing hamstring flexibility lowered the number of overuse injuries of lower limbs in military basic training (Hartig and Henderson 1999).

Flexibility is joint-specific. Some joints of an individual can have a flexibility greater than average while some other joints can have less than average flexibility—the same person can have normal mobility in the hip joints but suffer from impingement of the shoulder, and one joint of any pair of joints may be more mobile than the other. Flexibility in a joint is the sum of joint mobility. It depends primarily on the shape of joint surfaces, the length and pliability of ligaments and joint capsules, the length or the compliance of muscles associated with that joint, and in the case of active movements—the ability to combine tensing of the moving muscles with loosening of the extended muscles. Flexibility also depends on your emotional state, on the temperature of your body, the time of day, on the warm-up, initial position of the exercise, rhythm of movements, preparatory tensing of your muscles, and on your strength (Marciniak 1991; Tumanyan and Kharatsidis 1998).

Warm-up exercises have a very specific effect on the flexibility of various joints. For example, jogging for five minutes prepares well for ankle stretches but is a poor preparation for trunk stretches. People who did not jog prior to trunk stretches improved trunk flexibility more than people who jogged (Williford et al. 1986). Jogging puts most stress on the muscles moving the ankles, and the ankles go through most of their range of motion, but during jogging the muscles of the trunk keep its movements to a minimum.

Flexibility, just like coordination, is affected by the emotions because of the connection between the cerebellum and the areas of the brain responsible for emotions. This becomes obvious when an athlete (or anyone, for that matter) attempts juggling, balancing, or stretching when emotionally upset. Flexibility increases during excitement (Wazny 1981b).

Some motor qualities are inborn, such as speed; others, such as balance, have to be developed at a certain age to reach an exceptional level. Flexibility is like strength and endurance, however, in that it can be brought to high levels by anybody and at any time in a person's life as long as the joint surfaces permit normal mobility (Wazny 1981b). Ozolin, a renowned Russian authority on sports training, says, "Flexibility improves from day to day, strength from week to week, speed from month to month, endurance from year to year" (Ozolin 1971). Outside of pathological cases, exceptional flexibility is not inborn and requires work. If a more than natural range of motion is needed—for example, more than 50 degrees of turn-out (external rotation) in a hip joint, which is desired in ballet—then it may be necessary to elongate ligaments of the joint (Reid 1988). The earlier one starts flexibility exercises the easier it is to stretch the ligaments of the hip. In the case of the hip joint, it is best to start before the age of 11, before the angulation of the neck of the thigh bone becomes stable and before the ligaments become stronger and tighter (Ryan and Stephens 1988). By the way, researchers, some using X-rays, have found that dancers' unusually large range of external rotation in the hip joint is due to stretched-out ligaments and not to an abnormal shape of their thigh bone, i.e., femoral retroversion (Reid 1988).

Caution: Flexibility can be worsened by spending most of your training time moving joints through a shortened range of motion, as with some basketball players who spend most of their playing time in a crouched position, neglect general exercises, and end up with shortened hip and knee flexors (Orlikowska 1991).

You can improve flexibility by doing exercises such as running, swimming, and lifting weights as long as your limbs go through the full range of motion (Tumanyan and Dzhanyan 1980; Williams et al. 1988). (Lifting heavy weights does not reduce flexibility as long as the exercises are done in the full range. Powerlifters who do deadlifts have a greater range of hip flexion than people who do not do deadlifts [Chang 1988]. Even the elderly can increase their flexibility as a result of strength training at the full range of motion, with resistance permitting 6–10 repetitions without straining—and without any additional stretching exercises [Barbosa et al. 2002].)

For resistance exercises to increase flexibility, they have to be performed along the same path as the movement in which the increase of range of motion is sought, with the muscles that limit the range of motion overcoming resistance when stretched in every repetition. Resistance exercises for increasing flexibility have to look like stretches, in other words, but with the active movement done in the opposite direction and against resistance. The amount of resistance must be such as to permit the full range of motion in most repetitions of the exercise, of course. For example, to increase shoulder flexibility, do strength exercises from a stretched position, with resistance light enough to stretch the exercised muscles without danger of overstretching or of wrenching the shoulder (Platonov and Fesenko 1990). Resistance exercises may cause loss of flexibility if the

- muscles to be stretched are not the prime movers in the exercise,

- exercises are done along a different path than that in which range of motion is to be increased, or

- resistance is too heavy to permit the full range of motion.

Even static passive stretches done for 30 seconds before and after the resistance exercises may not offset this effect, as shown in the elderly by Girouard and Hurley (1995).

Not all athletes can always lift weights or run with long strides to move their legs through a full range of motion, though. At some stages of training, these exercises can interfere with the development of their sport-specific form. Properly chosen stretching exercises are less time- and energy-consuming than such indirect methods as lifting weights or running.

Apart from increasing the range of movement in your joints, stretching has other functions in your workout. At the beginning of the workout, some dynamic stretches can be good warm-up exercises. At the end of it, as a part of the cool-down, stretching facilitates recovery. It regulates muscular tension and relieves muscle spasms (deVries 1961). After stretching, blood flow in muscles is improved.

Relaxed static stretches relieve muscle cramps. Cramps happen to excessively tensed muscles, especially to chronically used muscles (Miles and Clarkson 1994), which is why they are relieved by passive stretching of the cramped muscles or by tensing their antagonists. (Prolonged profuse sweating may result in such electrolyte imbalance as to cause cramps too, but then more than just a stretch is needed to relieve them.)

Anatomy, physiology, and flexibility

Skeletal muscle consists of many muscle fibers (cells) arranged in parallel bundles. Muscle cells can grow in diameter by increasing the thickness and number of myofibrils, and in length by forming additional sarcomeres—the contractile elements of a muscle cell, lined end to end within each myofibril. Muscle cells have the ability to contract, and if relaxed, are very extensible. When a muscle contracts, two kinds of protein (actin and myosin) in the sarcomeres of its cells slide along one another. In the body, a muscle can be contracted to 70% or stretched to 130% of its normal resting length (Vander, Sherman, and Luciano 2001). "Normal resting length" is the length that the muscle takes up in the body in a typical resting attitude. Outside the body, the muscle can be contracted to 60% of its length and stretched more than 130%. As a muscle is stretched beyond its resting length, its force of contraction gradually drops, nearing zero at 200% of resting length (Wilmore and Costill 1999). Muscle contracts with greatest force at its normal resting length.

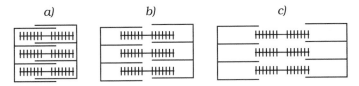

Amount of overlap of actin and myosin in a sarcomere—the contractile element of a muscle cell—a) contracted, b) resting, and c) stretched

When a muscle is stretched, the sarcomeres in the middle of the muscle fibers are more elongated than the sarcomeres at the ends of the muscle fibers (Goldspink 1968).

Exercises in which muscles tense as they are being stretched, for example, eccentric tensions and contract-relax stretches, cause changes in the muscle fibers that indicate an addition of new sarcomeres and thus lengthening the muscle fibers (Fridén 1984;

Handel et al. 1997; Lieber and Fridén 2000). So far, the actual increase in the serial sarcomere number has been shown in rats that did eccentric exercise (Lieber and Fridén 2000).

Research suggests that the bigger the muscles around a joint, the greater is the passive resistance to movement throughout the range of motion (Magnusson et al. 1997; Chleboun et al. 1997). This passive resistance can be decreased very effectively by continuous movements, such as dynamic stretches or resistance exercises done throughout the full range of motion (McNair et al. 2001; McNair and Stanley 1996; Wilson et al. 1992). Resistance training of calf muscles (resistance 70% of 1RM, 5 sets of 10 reps for 8 weeks) without stretching, for example, increases passive resistance to movement throughout the range of motion, but adding static stretching avoids this increase (Kubo et al. 2002a). Isometric strength exercises, if they are the sole mode of strength training, increase the hamstring's passive resistance throughout the range of motion, even when done together with passive static stretches (Klinge et al. 1997). A rational strength training is never limited to a single type of exercise, however, so this effect of isometric exercises (detrimental for some athletes) is offset by the influence of all the other types of exercises. For example, stretching and doing resistance exercises throughout the full range of motion lowers the stiffness of muscle-tendon unit (Wilson et al. 1992).

A *fibrous connective tissue sheath* (epimysium) encases the whole muscle. Bundles of muscle cells and even single cells are also surrounded by the same tissue (perimysium and endomysium). The tension generated by muscle cells is transferred to the fibers of connective tissue.

Tendons are cordlike extensions of this tissue. Collagen fibers, a major element of fibrous connective tissue, have great strength, little extensibility, and no ability to contract. These fibers are arranged in wavy bundles allowing motion until the slack of these bundles is taken up. Extension of a tendon beyond four percent of its length breaks cross-links between collagen fibers and starts irreversible deformation. Further extension, beyond eight percent of the tendon's length, weakens the tendon as more cross-links break until it eventually ruptures (Renström and Johnson 1986). With age, molecules of collagen change by becoming more rigid, which is reflected in general body stiffness. An improper use of isometric or eccentric tensions can put too much stress on muscle cells and collagen fibers, damaging them and causing delayed onset muscle soreness.

Muscle fibers   Collagen fibers

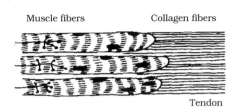

Tendon

Collagen fibers surrounding muscle fibers at their junction with the tendon

The stiffer the tendons, the better use of elastic energy in stretch-shorten cycle movements, provided you have the required range of motion (Kubo et al. 1999). If your range of motion is less than that required for taking full advantage of the stretch-shorten cycle, then it may be beneficial for you to increase the range of motion at the cost of lowering the stiffness of involved muscles and tendons (Wilson et al. 1992). Doing dynamic resistance training together with static stretching gives the benefits of increased tendon stiffness and increased reuse of elastic energy in a stretch-shorten cycle, without changing or increasing the passive resistance to the stretch (Kubo et al. 2002a).

Isometric strength training increases the stiffness of tendons and the longer the isometric contractions the greater the increase in stiffness (Kubo et al. 2001b; Kubo et al. 2001a).

You can permanently elongate tendons and connective tissue sheaths, with minimal structural weakening by low-force but long-duration stretching with temperatures of the tendons at more than 103°F. To increase the amount of permanent elongation, you maintain this stretch while tendons and sheaths cool down. This fits the description of a relaxed stretch done after the main part of your workout during the cool-down, with this qualifier: the stretch must be at the range of motion at which muscle fibers pose less resistance than the fibrous connective tissue.

Resistance exercises with movements of maximal amplitude, developing both strength and flexibility, are an effective means of increasing length and extensibility of tendons and connective tissue sheaths of muscles (Platonov 1997).

The *joint capsule* is a connective tissue sleeve that completely surrounds each movable joint. Immobilization for a few weeks causes chemical changes in the collagen fibers of the joint capsule that will restrict your flexibility.

The *ligaments* holding your joints together are made primarily of collagen fibers. They have more elastic fibers, made of the protein elastin, than do tendons. Stretching ligaments leads to loose-jointedness and can be effectively applied only with children. In adults, an age-related increase in the rigidity of collagen fibers makes any stretches aimed at elongating ligaments hazardous. When children stretch ballistically or statically, their muscles do not contract as strongly as an adult's, and their softer ligaments can be stretched (Raczek 1991). If a ligament is stretched more than six percent of its normal length, it tears. There is no need to stretch ligaments to perform even the most spectacular gymnastic or karate techniques. The normal range of motion is sufficient. Stretching ligaments destabilizes joints and thus may cause osteoarthritis (Beighton et al. 1983).

> One can have tight ligaments and good muscle flexibility or loose ligaments and poor muscle flexibility (Krivickas and Feinberg 1996).

Bone is a dynamic, living tissue made of collagen fibers associated with crystals of calcium and phosphorus. Exercises can change the density and shape of bones. The forms of joint surfaces, covered by a glasslike, smooth and elastic cartilage, also change in the long-term process of exercise, e.g., dynamic stretching or lifting weights. Depending on the amount of stress (exercise, for example), bones and joints can adapt to it or be destroyed by it.

Tests of flexibility potential

Here are simple tests you can do to see if the structure of your joints and the length of ligaments will not keep you from doing splits.

Front split. If the angle between the front and rear leg is less than 180 degrees with the front leg straight, flex the knee of your front leg and see what happens.

Front split with front leg straight

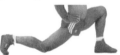

Deep lunge. The knee of the front leg is flexed and the angle between thighs is 180 degrees.

If you started to stretch past the age when elongating ligaments was feasible, you probably have difficulty touching the ground with the front thigh of the rear leg in this split. What keeps you from doing this is usually not a muscle, but a ligament (lig. iliofemorale) running in front of your hip joint. It is tightened by an extension of the hip (posterior tilting of the pelvis or moving the thigh to the back while keeping the pelvis straight). Flexing the hip (tilting the pelvis forward or moving the thigh to the front) relaxes this ligament. To achieve a nice, flat front split you need to stretch the hamstring of the front leg and the muscles of the lower back so you can tilt the pelvis forward while keeping the trunk upright.

To make sure that the muscles (hip flexors) pulling your thigh forward are not exceptionally short, do this test: Lie on a table, on your back, with your lower legs hanging over the edge. Pull one leg, with its knee flexed, toward your chest. Keep your back flat on the table. If the other leg, left lying on the table, is lifted by this movement before the angle between your thighs reaches 120 degrees, your iliopsoas (hip flexor) needs some stretching.

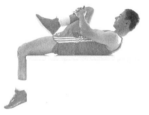

Iliopsoas length test

Side split. A person unable to do a complete split can bring one of the thighs into the position it would have in relation to the hip in the split, or at least get it much closer to this position than when spreading both legs at the same time. No muscles run from one leg to another. If you can do one half of the split, only the reflexive contraction of the muscles (and not the ligaments, or the muscles' connective tissue sheaths) prevents you from doing a complete split with equal ease. People with thick thigh bones and large and broad pelvises may not have enough range of motion in the hip joint to position their leg as shown in the following test and so cannot do a complete side split (Kapandji 1987).

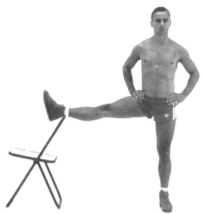

If you think that the structure of your hips will not let you do side splits, try this test. The leg resting on the chair is in the position it would have in a split.

One more test of the potential to do a side split—it is not as comprehensive as the preceding test, but it is informative nonetheless.

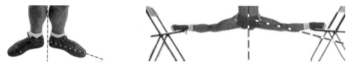

Outside rotation of the thigh in first ballet position. Nearly 90 degrees of turnout of the foot are achieved by 50 to 70 degrees of external rotation at the hip, plus about 20 degrees of external rotation at the knee and ankle (Reid 1988; Ryan and Stephens 1988). Note the relation of the angle (less than 90 degrees from the centerline) in this position, to the angle (less than 180 degrees) between the thighs in a side split.

The amount of outside rotation of the femur in the hip decides the quality of your side split (Kushner et al. 1990). This rotation is limited by the length of the ligaments of your hip joints, by the muscles that rotate the thigh inside, and in a few cases by the configuration of thigh bones.

Normally adductors pull the thigh inward and rotate it outward, but if the thigh is rotated outward as much as it takes to do a side split or a first ballet position, adductors also help to rotate it inward (Geselevich 1976), which means that, in addition to being stretched by abduction, adductors are also stretched by extreme outside rotation and can thus limit this rotation.

Note that in doing a side split you not only spread your legs sideways, but also you tilt your pelvis forward (the same way as when you lean forward so your trunk is parallel to the floor, pushing your buttocks to the rear) and rotate your thighs outward.

In a side split with the feet pointing up, you tilt your pelvis a little but rotate the thighs maximally outward. In a side split with the feet pointing forward, you tilt your pelvis strongly forward, and your thighs rotate outward as they are spread apart. The alignment of the hips and thighs in both types of the side split is the same. You cannot do this split without some combination of rotating your thighs outward and tilting your pelvis forward. Spreading the legs without these additional movements twists and tightens the ligaments of the hip and jams the tops of the necks of your thigh bones against the cartilage collar *(labrum acetabulare)* at the upper edge of your hip socket. It may also—if the angle between the neck and the shaft of the thigh bone is less than 135° *(coxa vara)*—jam the greater trochanters against the hip bone above the joint socket. Stretching the ligaments at the front and bottom of the hip joint (iliofemoral and pubofemoral ligaments) lets the head of the thigh bone slip partially downward out of the joint socket during abduction. This permits a greater angle of abduction before the neck of the thighbone contacts the upper edge of the joint socket (Ciszek and Smigielski 1997). The downside is a less stable hip joint.

> This jamming of either the neck of the thigh into the cartilage or, in the case of people with *coxa vara*, of the greater trochanters against the hip bones is the cause of pain and limits sideways movement in both the side split and the raising side kick.

The forward tilt of the pelvis (hip flexion) unwinds all capsular ligaments of the hip, among them the pubofemoral ligament, which resists abduction and outward rotation, and the iliofemoral ligament, which resists outward rotation (Kapandji 1987). Both the tilt and the outward rotation of the thigh reposition the socket of the hip joint in relation to the neck of the thigh bone so the brim of the joint cavity is faced with the flat frontal surface of the thigh-neck (the neck of the thigh bone is flattened front-to-back) and the greater trochanter faces the space behind the joint socket (Ciszek and Smigielski 1997). See figures 4–6 in Appendix A, pages 185–186. (A similar ease-of-movement technique happens in the shoulder joint—you can move your arm a little further up sideways without moving your shoulder blade if you rotate your arm outward so the greater tuberosity of the arm bone does not hit the acromion or the ligament that stretches between the acromion and coracoid process.)

Another way of finding the correct alignment is to use the horse-riding stance as the initial position for your isometric stretches leading to the side split. The horse-riding stance averts irritation of the upper brim of the hip socket and the resulting pain above the hip joint. Just make sure that your stance is correct, with your thighs parallel to the floor at any width, toes pointing forward, and chest up.

Starting position   *End position*   *End position*
for a side split   *in a side split* *in a side split*
with feet   *with feet*   *with feet*
pointing forward   *pointing forward* *pointing up*

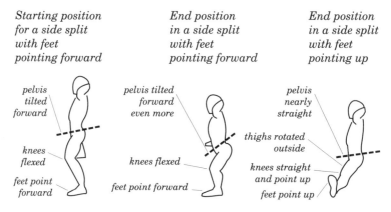

Correct alignment of thighs and pelvis in side splits

> To sum it all up, you cannot do the side split without combining the outward rotation of your thighs with a forward tilt of your pelvis. And yes, there are people whose hip joints may not have enough range in these motions to permit doing a side split. Those are the people with thick thigh bones and large and broad pelvises (Kapandji 1987).

In the examples of joint mobility tests on pages 108 and 110, relieving the tension of the muscles around the joint increases its range of motion. If you can perform these tests of joint structure and ligament length, this means that only muscular tension prevents you from doing splits. Muscular tension has two components: the tension actively generated by the contractile elements of stimulated muscle fibers; and the passive tension present even in an inactive, denervated muscle, due mainly to the connective tissues associated with the muscle and, to a much lesser degree, the microstructure of myofibrils (resting tension). Some authors (M. J. Alter, H. A. deVries, S. A. Sölveborn) declare the connective tissue tension to be the main factor restricting flexibility. They advocate slow static stretching, even in a warm-up, as if muscles were pieces of fabric to be elongated to a desired size. In the muscle stretched to well over 100% of its resting length, however, the resting tension is a small fraction of the tension due to active contraction. Eventually, at approximately 120% of a muscle's resting length, the two components of muscle tension contribute about equally to total tension (Schottelius and Senay 1956). (Remember that 130% of resting length is usually the maximum stretch of a muscle in the body.) At greater lengths the resting (passive) tension increases while the active tension, generated by contracting muscle fibers, decreases.

Recent research gives conflicting answers as to what limits flexibility or range of motion—neural factors or the mechanical properties of a muscle with its connective tissue. In the case of single stretches of the hamstrings Magnusson et al. (1998) conclude that either a slow dynamic passive stretch or a static passive stretch increases range of motion "by increasing stretch tolerance [a neural factor] while the viscoelastic characteristics [mechanical properties] of the muscle remain unaltered." Halbertsma et al. (1996) showed a similar result after one 10-minute session of static passive stretches. In another study Magnusson et al. (1996a) showed that Proprioceptive Neuromuscular Facilitation (PNF) stretching of hamstrings increased range of motion more than passive static stretching and concluded that PNF stretching altered stretch perception (again, a neural factor). This differs from the conclusion of McHugh et al. (1998) that flexibility is determined by mechanical properties of muscles rather than by neural factors because in the case of slow static stretches of the hamstring, with muscles of the thigh completely relaxed, "seventy-nine percent of variability in maximum . . . range of motion could be explained by the passive mechanical response to stretch."

Long-term studies are similarly ambiguous. Magnusson et al. (1996b) conclude that three weeks of slow static stretching of hamstring muscles increased range of motion as "a consequence of increased stretch tolerance [a neural factor] . . . rather than a change in mechanical or viscoelastic properties of the muscle" because the passive resistance to stretch did not change. Also similar was the conclusion of Halbertsma and Goeken (1994) after four weeks of passive static stretching of hamstrings. In contrast, Kubo et al. (2002b) concluded that three weeks of static passive stretching of the calf muscles lowered passive resistance to stretch by affecting the connective tissue in the muscle. Three weeks of stretching the calves using the contract-relax method also resulted in lowering the passive resistance to stretch in an experiment by Toft et al. (1989). Wilson et al. (1992) showed that eight weeks of stretching chest muscles increased flexibility and reduced stiffness of musculotendinous unit—probably by reducing stiffness of the tendons.

None of these studies shows with absolute certainty that flexibility is decisively determined either by the neural factors or by the mechanical properties of the muscle, especially of its connective tissue.

There are certainly arguments for the considerable role of the nervous system in determining flexibility. For instance, three different types of stretches increase the static range of motion in varying degrees, both in a single stretch as well as in several sessions of stretching (Holt et al. 1970; Tanigawa 1972). So, a contract-relax stretch increases range of motion more than a static passive stretch, and a contract-relax-antagonist-contract stretch increases range of motion more than a contract-relax stretch (Etnyre and Abraham 1986a). These stretches differ in the utilization and sequence of muscle tensions—actions that affect the nervous regulation of stretched muscles. Further, Tanigawa (1972) showed that while the subjects who used contract-relax stretching for three weeks twice per week gained more range of motion than those doing passive stretches, they also lost more range during one week of not stretching. If connective tissue were the chief determinant of flexibility these different gains and losses with the two types of static stretches wouldn't make sense.

For practical purposes, as long as you feel your muscles contract in response to a stretch, it means that relaxing the muscles can improve your stretch and that you should concern yourself more with nervous regulation of your muscles' tension and less with your muscles' connective tissue.

The nervous system regulates tension and thus the length of your muscles by influencing the contractile element. (The illustration on page 115 sums up what follows.)

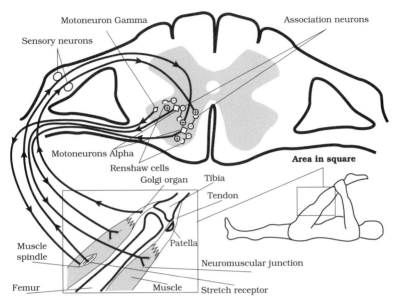

Structures and nerve pathways involved in control of a muscle at the level of its corresponding segment of spinal cord

Several nerve cells receive signals from and send signals to each muscle. Nerve cells receiving the signals are called sensory neurons. Directly, or through other neurons, they contact nerve cells that send signals to the muscles. The cells whose nerve fibers conduct signals to the muscles are called motoneurons. Their cell bodies are located in the spinal cord or in the brainstem. Other neurons contact and influence motoneurons. Some can stimulate the motoneurons, which causes a contraction of the muscle fibers innervated by them. Some can inhibit (block) motoneurons, causing a relaxation of muscle fibers. In movements, when the motoneurons of one set of muscles are stimulated, motoneurons of the muscles opposing them are inhibited. This is called *reciprocal inhibition.* It allows you to move.

Neurons causing contraction of muscles are called *motoneurons Alpha.* Doing dynamic stretches as a warm-up for a dynamic action requires stimulating motoneurons of the moving, contracting muscles in a way that is similar to the stimulation they will receive during the action. During static stretches those motoneurons are not stimulated in such a way.

Muscle spindles are embedded within a muscle at the midpoints of some muscle fibers. They consist of special kinds of muscle fibers (intrafusal muscle fibers) that can contract only at their ends. At their center are the stretch receptors. There are two kinds of stretch receptors: one responding only to the magnitude of the stretch; and another that responds to both the magnitude and the speed of stretching (Bishop 1982). Stretch receptors in a stretched muscle send signals that reach a motoneuron Alpha and cause it to send impulses to the muscle. For example, when a muscle is stretched by tapping its tendon as in testing the knee-jerk reflex, receptors in the spindles send impulses that reach motoneurons Alpha, stimulating the contraction of this muscle and its synergists, or cooperating muscles. The same impulse, sent by stretch receptors, inhibits muscles antagonistic to it, and so your leg kicks. This knee-jerk reflex is an example of a myotatic or stretch reflex. A quick stretch causes a contraction preventing further stretching. This contraction lowers the stimulation of the spindles.

During an isometric contraction the frequency of signals from the muscle spindle is decreased (Bishop 1982; Orlikowska 1991; Vander, Sherman, and Luciano 2001). This may be the neural mechanism behind your not feeling stretching when you are tensing a muscle stretched below the pain threshold, such as during the tensing phase of an isometric stretch. This effect, together with what happens to a muscle as it is stretched and tensed, may also explain why it is easier to increase range of motion after an isometric tension than without it. As a stretched muscle is tensed, the sarcomeres in the middle of muscle fibers shorten and stretch the sarcomeres at the fibers' ends together with the fibrous connective tissue in series with them, picking up the slack. Relaxing after such tension releases the slack and this could be why you can extend the range of motion further before feeling a new stretch limit.

The *Golgi organs* are located in the tendon at its junction with the muscle and detect changes in tension generated either by contracting a muscle or by stretching it. The most effective stimulus for Golgi organs is an active muscle contraction (Houk et al. 1971). Each Golgi organ is connected with from five to twenty-five muscle fibers. As the contracting muscle pulls on the tendon it causes the Golgi organs to fire impulses in relation to the force of contraction (Bishop 1982). These impulses activate association neurons, which then send their impulses to inhibit the motoneurons Alpha of the contracting muscle. This stops the flow of impulses from the motoneurons Alpha to the muscle. (This is the usual explanation for the mechanism of PNF [Proprioceptive Neuromuscular Facilitation] and isometric stretching.) The Golgi organs may also influence motoneurons Gamma (Bishop 1982).

Renshaw cells are small nerve cells located close to the motoneurons Alpha. They are connected through synapses with motoneurons and are activated by the impulses that these motoneurons send to muscle fibers. Renshaw cells through their axons synapse back both on the motoneurons that activate them and on others. Impulses from the Renshaw cells inhibit motoneurons. This circuit regulates the frequency of impulses received by muscles and keeps them from making contractions that are too strong. Renshaw cells are connected with both the small (tonic) motoneurons Alpha innervating slow-twitch muscle fibers and with the large (phasic) motoneurons Alpha innervating fast-twitch muscle fibers. Renshaw cells are more strongly excited by impulses from phasic motoneurons activated in voluntary contractions than by impulses from tonic motoneurons, but when excited they inhibit tonic motoneurons, which are most responsive to the stretch reflex, much more so than are phasic ones (Bishop 1982). This is another possible explanation of PNF and isometric stretching.

There are neural circuits and pathways that may cause lessened resistance to stretch, more formally called *postcontractive reflex depression.* Postcontractive reflex depression follows a strong voluntary contraction of the muscle. It permits a greater range of motion increase than stretching without a preceding contraction. No matter what the exact cause of lessening the resistance to stretch, the resistance is smallest immediately upon relaxation following a contraction of the muscles about to be stretched. (Moore and Kukulka [1991] have shown that reflexes are weakest within the first second of relaxation after a contraction of the muscle and then recover to nearly 70% of their normal values by the fifth second. This may be why your stretch is easiest within the first second after the end of a contraction.) Resistance to stretching can be reduced even more by immediately following the relaxation of the stretched muscles with contraction of their antagonists (Etnyre and Abraham 1986a; Etnyre and Abraham 1986b; Etnyre and Abraham 1988).

Motoneurons Gamma are located in the spinal cord, close to motoneurons Alpha. These neurons regulate the tension of intrafusal fibers in muscle spindles, so that if the whole muscle is shortened, the spindle can adjust and still be able to detect changes in muscle length. There are two types of motoneurons Gamma: static and dynamic. Static Gamma determine length sensitivity of receptors in the muscle spindle with little effect on velocity sensitivity. Dynamic Gamma determine velocity sensitivity with little effect on length sensitivity (Bishop 1982).

The brain, through its pathways of nerve fibers conducting impulses downwards, similarly affects motoneurons Alpha and

Gamma, but the Gamma are more sensitive. Static Gamma motoneurons, which regulate the muscle spindles' detection of the magnitude of a stretch, are stimulated by the cold center and inhibited by the heat center in your hypothalamus (Bishop 1982). Static motoneurons Gamma are thus easier to activate when your body temperature is low and so your flexibility worsens then. (When cold is applied locally, for example, to a single muscle group, the effect may be opposite—the stretching may become easier. This is because local cooling reduces the sensitivity of muscle spindles but not of the Golgi organs [Meeusen and Lievens 1986; Strzelczyk 1996].)

Mental stress, pain, anxiety, and fear, thanks to these same descending pathways, activate motoneurons Gamma, which increase the stretch reflex, thus making you less flexible (Sölveborn 1989). This is one more reason not to do static passive stretches during a warm-up when you may be excited or even anxious about the challenging activities ahead. (The ways of warming up to deal with prestart anxiety and prestart apathy are described in the book *Science of Sports Training*.)

Descending pathways, motoneurons Gamma, spindle muscle fibers, stretch receptors (in a particular spindle), sensory neurons (innervating a particular spindle), and a motoneuron Alpha are collectively called the Gamma loop. The Gamma loop activity measures and influences the length and tension of a muscle. Thanks to this loop, the same weight can be supported by different lengths of a muscle or, the same length can support different weights. The Gamma loop regulates the sensitivity of muscle spindles. If, because of lowered tonus, an insufficient amount of impulses comes from stretch receptors, the Gamma loop compensates, making the muscle spindles shorter. This may be why people experience stiffness upon first awakening.

Your kinesthetic, or muscle and joint, sense is served by more than the already-described kinds of receptors (muscle spindles and Golgi organs). There are receptors of pain, pressure, joint position, and movement located in the joint capsules, ligaments, tendons, muscles and their fasciae, and in skin.

The combined input from all the receptors influences your reflexive reactions to changes in your body position and muscular tension. Your actual reflexes are never as simple as the oversimplified description of a knee-jerk. Usually the whole body responds to any stimulus. Recall the test (see page 110) where you could see whether the bones and ligaments of your hips would let you do a side split. There is no muscle or ligament running from one thigh to another, yet, even if you have passed the test, you cannot do a complete side split without some training. When you spread both legs at the same time, the reflexive contraction of the muscles, on both sides of the body, gets in your way. Reflexes serve useful purposes in normal circumstances and, when your legs slide sideways, the tension of the adductors and their synergists on both sides of the body is needed to maintain upright posture.

So much for the reflexive regulation of muscular tension. Now consider the brain's role in control of muscular tension through either stimulating or inhibiting the motoneurons.

Some of the nerve fibers conducting kinesthetic information go to the cerebellum where, without your being aware of it, your tonus, coordination, and balance are regulated. Other fibers go to the cerebral cortex, the outer layer of the brain, which contains higher centers that interpret and correlate sensory data. These fibers provide you with sensory data you are conscious of: the data you feel. The neurons located in the cerebral cortex contact motoneurons through the descending pathways.

Descending pathways consist of nerve fibers originating in the cerebral cortex and ending in the spinal cord. These fibers either directly contact the motoneurons Alpha, Gamma, or association neurons in the spinal cord (the direct descending pathways), or first synapse with neurons in nerve centers below the cortex and in the cerebellum. In turn, those neurons eventually synapse on motoneurons Alpha, Gamma, or on association neurons (the multineuronal descending pathways). The direct pathways govern precise, voluntary movements. Through conscious decisions to make certain movements or to contract groups of muscles, you can override some of your reflexes.

The multineuronal descending pathways are responsible for the control of rapid movements, postural mechanisms, the coordination of simultaneous movements of locomotion, and the coordination of fine voluntary movements with postural mechanisms. The connection between the cerebellum and the areas of the brain governing emotions (hippocampus, amygdala, septal areas), makes muscular tonus and coordination dependent on emotions, and vice versa (Grochmal 1986). Mental stress increases amplitude and decreases the frequency of muscle tremor possibly by increasing the gain of the stretch reflex (Growdon et al. 2000).

Yoga uses this connection. Yoga exercises (asanas) do not use tension in a stretched position. By holding relaxed muscles in a position just short of pain and reflexive contraction, Yogis (in a long-term process) gradually lower the sensitivity of the mechanisms regulating the tension and length of the muscles. Yoga stretches seem to be a litmus test, or a sort of biofeedback monitor, telling the practitioner how proper (from a Yoga point of view) his or her state of mind is.

Practical conclusions for sports training

Muscle fibers are very stretchable but in the muscle they are connected with the less stretchable fibrous connective tissue. This fact is used to explain the loss of flexibility solely as a result of the shortening of the connective tissue in and around the muscles. Such shortening can be caused by lack of movement or by exercising regularly within less than a full range of motion.

But there is more to it than that. Different stretching methods bring about differing results: dynamic stretching improves dynamic flexibility (dynamic range of motion and resistance to stretching throughout the range of motion); static stretching improves static flexibility (static range of motion) and, to a limited extent, dynamic flexibility (Moscov and Lacourse 1992). Continuous movements decrease resistance to stretching throughout the range of motion more effectively than static stretching, while static stretching more effectively increases the range of motion and decreases the amount of force needed to hold a stretch or tension in a static position (McNair and Stanley 1996; McNair et al. 2001). Furthermore the stretching method you choose—ballistic (bobbing up and down in a stretch, not advisable), static relaxed, or isometric—affects the amount of time to reach the current maximum in each stretching session and time to achieve desired results (Etnyre and Abraham 1986a; Holt et al. 1970; Lucas and Koslow 1984; Sady et al. 1982; Tanigawa 1972). After exercises increasing range of motion through active movements (for example, dynamic stretches or static active stretches), the increase of flexibility lasts longer than after passive stretching (Starzynski and Sozanski 1999). The possible changes in connective tissues resulting from stretching by any of these methods do not explain all the differences. These differences are most likely the result of the way a given kind of exercise acts upon the nervous system.

Muscles are usually long enough to allow for a full range of motion permitted by the structures of joints. It is the nervous control of their tension, however, that has to be reset for the muscles to show their full length. This is the most likely explanation why ten minutes of dynamic stretching in the morning lets you display your full range of motion in dynamic movements later in a day without a warm-up. Regularly repeating movements that do not use a full range of motion in the joints (e.g., bicycling, certain exercises of Olympic weightlifting, standard push-ups on the floor), however, sets the nervous control of length and tension in the muscles at the values repeated most often or most strongly and so diminishes the range of motion (Orlikowska 1991). Immediately after a fatiguing jog or a slow run in which the athlete's legs moved at a reduced range of motion, both dynamic and static flexibility of the hips and knees are temporarily diminished. It seems to be the result of increased sensitivity of stretch receptors—neural compensation for the effects of fatigue on the muscles' contractions. While this compensatory mechanism is supposed to work in all fatigue-inducing and high-tension exercises (Hayes 1976) it does not cause such a drastic reduction of flexibility if in these exercises limbs move through their full range of motion. So, displaying your full range of motion while fatigued (but not extremely fatigued!) after doing heavy deep squats is easier than after a long run.

The other factor in diminishing the range of motion, relevant to many successive workouts, is shortening of muscle fibers (loss of serial sarcomeres) in the muscles that work only over a reduced range of motion (Williams et al. 1988). Eastern European coaches will not let their gymnasts ride bicycles as a means of endurance training, for example, even though they seem to have all the flexibility they need.

Strenuous workouts slightly damage the fibers of connective tissue in the muscles. Usually these micro-tears heal in a day or two, but a loss of flexibility is supposedly caused by these fibers healing at a shorter length. To prevent this, some physiologists recommend static stretching after strength workouts. All this sounds very good, but the same gymnasts who are kept from bicycling, run with maximal accelerations to improve their specific endurance. Such running is a strenuous, intensive strength effort for leg muscles, but in fast running, lower limb muscles work through a full range of motion in the hip and knee joints, and because of that there is no adverse effect on flexibility. If connective tissue were a factor, then stretching after a workout would be enough and these gymnasts could ride bicycles with the same result. The situation with standard push-ups is very similar. If you do a couple of hundred a day, on the floor, so the muscles of your chest, shoulders, and arms contract from a shortened position, no amount of static stretching will make you a baseball pitcher or a javelin thrower.

There are two types of stretch receptors, one detecting the magnitude and speed of stretching, the other detecting magnitude only. Sensitivity of each type of receptor is determined by the respective type of motoneurons Gamma (through regulating tension of either type of intrafusal fibers in muscle spindles [Bishop 1982; McArdle, Katch, and Katch 1996]). This may explain why flexibility training is speed-specific.

Static stretches improve static flexibility and dynamic stretches improve dynamic flexibility, which is why it does not make sense to use static stretches as a warm-up for dynamic action. There is considerable, but not complete, transfer from static to dynamic flexibility (Moscov and Lacourse 1992).

Dynamic stretching by movements similar to the task—for example, leg raises before kicking, lunges before fencing, arm swings before playing tennis—done with gradually increasing range and speed of motion facilitate neural pathways that will be used in the task. (*Facilitation* means increased excitability of neurons by means of repetitive use or the accumulation of impulses arriving from other neurons.) These movements of gradually increasing range and speed of motion require muscular contractions increasingly similar to those of the task (kick, fencing attack, serve). These contractions cause arterioles and capillaries in the working muscles to dilate in proportion to the force of contraction (McArdle, Katch, and Katch 1996). Flexibility improves with an increased flow of blood in stretched muscles (Wazny 1981b).

Static stretches do not facilitate these pathways, do not prepare the nervous system and blood vessels in muscles for the dynamic task. You even sweat differently when warming up with dynamic actions than when doing static stretches. During dynamic exercises you sweat all over and your sweat is hot. During static stretching you sweat little, mainly on the face. This tells you that static stretching is a poor warm-up.

Flexibility training is also position-specific. Research done by Nicolas Breit (1977), comparing the effects of stretching in the supine and the erect position, shows that:

a) subjects who trained in an erect position tested better in this position than subjects who trained in a supine but tested in an erect position.

b) greater gains were recorded for both groups in a supine test position than in an erect test position. The subjects tested in the erect position had to overcome an extra amount of tension in the muscles they stretched because of the reflexes evoked by standing and bending over.

You can use the postcontractive reflex depression or increased "stretchability" (lower resistance to a stretch following a strong contraction), caused by any of the explained mechanisms by contracting a muscle before relaxing and stretching it. This increases the amount of possible stretch. The contraction can be short—3 seconds may be enough (Nelson and Cornelius 1991). The stretch has to be done within five seconds of relaxation after contraction and preferably in the first second.

After reaching a maximal stretch (maximal for you at a given stage of your training), tensing the muscle to hold this position longer than the few seconds typically used to cause the postcontractive relaxation further increases your static strength in this maximal range of motion or stretch. A strength increase in extreme ranges of motion (caused by systematic isometric stretching or resistance exercises in a full range of motion) seems to be a result, at least to a degree, of the longitudinal growth of muscle fibers. Long-term exercise, in which human muscles tense as they are stretched, causes changes in the muscle fibers that indicate their lengthening through adding new sarcomeres (Fridén 1984). Handel et al. (1997) conducted a study in which athletes did contract-relax stretches (stretches with isometric contractions) for eight weeks and showed changes in strength displayed throughout the range of motion that indicated longitudinal growth of muscle fibers by the addition of sarcomeres. The opposite happens when exercises are done exclusively at a reduced range of motion—there is loss of sarcomeres and muscles shorten (Williams et al. 1988).

Strong muscles tense less than weak ones to support the same load (Moritani and deVries 1979; Ploutz et al. 1994). The strong muscles can be more elongated while still comfortably overcoming resistance. In the muscles of strong people, who regularly overcome high resistance, motor units (several muscle fibers and a nerve cell activating them) synchronize their action even when overcoming low resistance (Hayes 1976). This may be why athletes whose thigh muscles are strong enough to slide up from a split to standing upright can slide down into a split with less muscle tension and resistance to the stretch than weaker persons. Perhaps when all motor units tense together even moderately, the stretch reflex is more depressed than if only some motor units were tensing very hard, either because of stimulating a greater number of Golgi organs, or because of the mechanical effect on all the muscle fibers and the connective tissue in series with them.

As people age, changes occur in their muscles that are associated with a decrease in strength and flexibility—loss of muscle mass and increased stiffness of fibrous connective tissue. Does that mean that the elderly cannot effectively use isometric stretches? No, it does not— because these changes can be offset by strength training—even in very old age (Fiatarone et al. 1990; Evans 1999). As long as your joints are not deformed and permit normal range of motion, and there is no contraindication for strength training, you can benefit from isometric stretches. What range of motion you can achieve and how fast depends on the initial level of your flexibility and strength. If your muscles are long enough for splits (you can check it with tests shown on pages 108 and 110), you might be able to make them strong enough to support you in a split—even though gains in absolute terms may come more slowly than in the case of young people.

Coordination and flexibility depend on your emotions too, because of the connection between the cerebellum and the areas of the brain responsible for emotions. Try juggling, balancing, or stretching when you are upset!

The opening caution you read is worth repeating: Mental rigidity— the inability to abandon fixed ideas, a sign of low intelligence—is usually accompanied by a low level of physical flexibility—perhaps due to the connection between flexibility and coordination (Matveyev [Matveev] 1981), and coordination is considered a motor expression of intellect (Wazny 1981a).

Recap

The following factors are listed in order of their importance in improving flexibility.

- The greatest and fastest gains are made by resetting the nervous control of muscle tension and length.

- Special strength exercises can stimulate the muscle fibers to grow longer and elongate the fibrous connective tissue associated with the muscle.

- Stretching the ligaments and joint capsules and ultimately reshaping joint surfaces takes years and brings about the smallest amount of improvement (Matveyev [Matveev] 1981).

9. Questions and Answers on Stretching

These are typical questions from readers of this book. Among them may be just the type that you want to ask. Study the answers, and perhaps you will be able to apply them to your situation.

Does This Method Really Work? And How?

People who don't believe what they see ask the variations of the question "Is it truly possible . . . ?" because, I guess, they were not exposed to rational sports training.

Question: Is it truly possible to produce a permanent, instantly accessible flexibility that requires no warm-up or any other preparation?

Answer: Yes. Otherwise what is the point of practicing martial arts techniques such as high kicks if they require a warm-up? I personally know many athletes who can display much greater flexibility without a warm-up than what I show in this book. Of course, I can do everything that you see in this book also without a warm-up. If your coach or instructor cannot teach you how to have such flexibility, then it tells you something about his or her knowledge of human physiology and of the methodology of sports training.

Question: How long it takes to do full front and side splits using your book?

Answer: It depends on your strength and initial flexibility. Some people reach splits within a month while others need several months.

Question: Why does the body have a natural tendency to prevent one from doing a split? I know that I have the ability to do a split because when I do side lunges (one leg extended and one leg pulled in, supporting my body) I can do a "half-split." That is, I can fully abduct (extend to the side) one leg till my pelvis hits the floor—but with my other leg pulled in underneath me. I can do this with both legs but not at the same time. Why does the nervous system have to be trained to allow for fully abducting both legs at the same time?

Answer: To find out more about the nervous system read about the reflexes in neurology textbooks or see pages 115–119 in this book.

Apart from your nervous system not being used to spreading both legs at the same time, your adductors may be weak. Weak adductors tense harder and stop your legs' sidewise movement earlier than strong adductors when sliding your legs apart in a straddle stance. The wider the angle between your legs, the less efficient is your adductors' leverage, and the harder they tense to keep the legs from sliding apart.

Question: I wonder about the results of your method in people past thirty years of age. I started taekwondo in my late 30s and currently I am 42 years old. I would like to know if it is possible for me to do the splits without injuring myself.

Answer: As long as your muscles are responsive to strength training (you feel they are getting stronger), they are also responsive to stretching. We have plenty of testimonials from people past their 30s saying and showing that they just achieved a full side split.

Question: Most of the stretches you show are practiced daily at my martial arts school. In fact most of them were taught to us in high school. Also, isometrics or dynamic tension is nothing new to this country. So why should your results be better?

Answer: It is not exercises alone that make my method effective. It is the way of arranging them in the proper sequence during a workout, during a day, and during a weekly cycle of workouts. Doing the same exercises in the wrong order reduces their effectiveness. I explain how various coordination, speed, strength, endurance, and flexibility exercises influence each other. Some exercises should follow each other and some should not.

Question: I practice karate and my teacher can lift a leg and hold it steady above his shoulder. Will your static active stretches let me achieve this type of strength so I can kick higher and with more power?

Answer: Yes and no. Static active flexibility exercises will help to develop your ability to lift and hold the leg but not to make your kicks more powerful. Specific strength for a kicker is the strength that lets you pack a wallop in a kick, not to hold a leg up! Specific strength for kicking is developed by kicking a heavy bag, kicking into layers of sponge, kicking with bungee cords attached to legs, and other dynamic exercises similar to kicking. Strength, just like flexibility, is specific to the speed of movement, its angle, and range of motion (McArdle, Katch, and Katch 1996).

Question: Do you have a schedule of what, when, and in which order stretches are done to achieve a full split? I have *Stretching Scientifically* but I think a specific routine would be better.

Answer: While the book does not give specific (specific for whom and when?) routines, it explains the principles of selecting and sequencing exercises so readers who studied chapters 2 and 7 know when to do what type of stretches depending on their needs and limitations.

Question: How do you get on those chairs?

Answer: One way is to stand on them when they are close to each other and then spread your legs with the chairs. Another way is to place the chairs so they are as far apart as your feet in a split and then do a handstand between them, lower your legs onto the chairs and push off the floor with your hands to assume the final position. When trying to learn this skill, you should start by using two books or small blocks of wood.

Question: How often should suspended splits be tried, and how do you maintain your strength and flexibility once you have achieved a suspended split?

Answer: Every time you can lift yourself off the floor while sitting in a split you are proving that you have enough strength to do a suspended split. I do not see any reason for most athletes ever to try an actual suspended split. I did it to catch your attention, but as far as strengthening legs goes there are many better and safer exercises.

Question: I have purchased [*Stretching Scientifically*] and your video *Secrets of Stretching*. While my side splits have improved, my front splits are still lacking. In my style of Chinese martial arts, we must be able to drop into front and side splits. I can slowly lower into a full side split, but if I try to drop into one I can only come within one foot of the floor. As for my front splits, I am stuck at less than six inches from the floor. What can I do to remedy this?

Answer: One of the ways of training for the ability to drop into splits is developing such strength as to be able to slide up from a split to a standing position. You already know the exercises you need for this purpose and the method of using them because they are shown on the video *Secrets of Stretching.*

Question: Are the side split and the front split independent or dependent? I mean that if I can't do a side split, I can't do a front split and vice versa. Can I do an isometric stretch for a side split only without developing my front split ability?

Answer: Flexibility is joint- and muscle-specific. One can be able to do a flat side split without being able to do a flat front split and vice versa. If your hip joints have normal mobility, then you can achieve sitting flat in both splits but only if you work on both of them. Isometric stretching for one of the splits will help somewhat with the other. There is some transfer of the training effect between the two splits because some muscles are stretched by both of them—but not to the same degree.

Body Alignment for Hip Stretches

Question: What is the difference between suspended side splits with toes pointing forward and with toes pointing upward?

Answer: The split with toes pointing forward stresses mainly the thigh adductors and requires less outside rotation of the hip joint than the split with toes pointing upward. The suspended split with toes pointing upward stresses your hamstrings in addition to thigh adductors and, for maintaining balance, requires greater outward rotation of the hip joint than the split with toes pointing forward.

Question: On page 64 you show a side split with toes pointing up. Why do you not describe how to gradually stretch into this position?

Answer: Because you can stretch for this split the same as for the one with toes pointing forward. Alignment of hips and thighs in both splits is the same, as is explained on pages 111 and 112.

Question: My goal is to do a complete side split with the toes pointing upward. Can I do isometric stretches with my heels on the floor and my toes pointing upward? Will this strengthen the correct muscles or will it throw my hips out of alignment for splits?

Answer: The safe isometric stretch for the side split with the toes pointing upward is shown on page 64.

Turning your toes up while sliding down into a side split without holding on to some firm support is asking for a muscle tear or worse (a joint capsule tear or a ligament sprain) because of having no control over the sliding legs and the precarious balance. (See the questions related to injuries on pages 165–171 for descriptions of outcomes with such a stretch.) The most vulnerable muscle seems to be the adductor magnus because in the toes-up position, abduction is combined with the external rotation of the thigh so the adductor magnus is stretched more than in the normal side split with soles of the feet on the ground.

Question: I have read *Stretching Scientifically* and find it helpful. I cannot do the side splits, however. I am beyond the starting position you show in your book, but not at a side split. I am not clear on the position of the feet. When going into a side split, should the soles of my feet remain planted on the ground, or should I allow the inner sides of my feet to be on the ground, which would result in the soles of my feet not being planted on the ground? When I allow the inner sides of my feet to be on the ground, my legs tend to bend at the knees, causing pain. How important is the position of the feet in the straddle position?

Answer: The position of your feet in the straddle stance (or the horse-riding stance) is important for reasons explained on page 62. Plant your feet as shown on pages 61 and 63, as long as you are in the horse-riding stance—however wide. When you spread your legs so wide that you are no longer in even the widest horse-riding stance, then your feet will turn and your weight will be supported by the insides of your lower legs and feet. When you are so low in the split that your weight is supported by the insides of your lower legs your knees should not hurt.

Question: In one of my Kung-Fu training sessions, I was told by a fellow student that practicing leg raises in the morning was good for flexibility. I tried it out only to find that I had pain in my knees and hips from trying it. After reading your book, I discovered that my hips were in the wrong place and I was keeping my leg too straight. Not surprisingly, the pain went away and I've started to make progress. My problem now is that when I'm in the wide horse-riding stance, I get pain in my knees. Could it be that I'm making a similar mistake and causing the pain?

Answer: Knee pain in the horse-riding stance may be caused by a wrong position of the feet (not pointing forward) and by doing too much too soon (stance too deep, standing too long). In the correct horse-riding stance you cannot have your legs straight.

Question: When I stand in *kiba dachi* (the horse-riding stance) and try to go lower I get a pain in my lower back and the only way to relieve this is to lean forward. Could you recommend any stretches to relieve the pain? Also I lose the strength to pinch the floor after a couple of cycles of tensing and spreading my legs.

When I do the side split, I can't do the split with toes pointing forward, I have to lean my whole upper body forward. If I try to do the split with toes pointing forward while keeping my body upright, I feel pain in the upper outside region of the thighs.

Answer: These problems are slightly different, but the answer is the same for both. A tendency for leaning forward when standing in a straddle stance is normal. You lean forward because your pelvis positions itself for greater range of hip abduction, but the weakness or inflexibility of your lower back (or both) keeps you from keeping your upper body upright as your pelvis tilts forward. How straight you can keep your trunk depends on the strength of your back erectors and alignment of your legs. Even at the lowest position in the split they should be aligned like the horse-riding stance. To develop flexibility and strength of your thighs, hips, and lower back in the horse-riding stance, start high and with feet only shoulder-width apart and gradually progress lower and then wider. If you want to make faster progress, do deep squats with weights. When doing these squats, stand with your feet a shoulder-width apart and try to keep your toes pointing forward.

Feeling pain in the outside of the hip joint results from not tilting the pelvis during abduction (sideways movement) of the thighs. Not having enough strength of the inner thighs for tensing them while standing firmly in the straddle stance ("pinching the floor") can be remedied by squats and exercises that specifically target inner thighs, such as the adductor flys and adductor pulldowns shown on the video *Secrets of Stretching*.

Question: I seem to be very tight in the hips so when I keep my back straight and tilt my pelvic forward I can't get as close to the floor as I can when I lean forward onto a small chair. Is this OK?

Answer: It is OK but it is better to develop the ability to stand in the proper horse-riding stance as the strength and flexibility of the thighs, hips, and spine comes in handy in other exercises. Also, when you lean on a chair in your isometric stretches you take the load off the thighs so you do not strengthen them as much as when they carry your whole weight.

Question: In my martial arts classes I have students who have started a little late in life (28–50). The majority of the adult students have moderate to severe hip pain or discomfort during kicking drills and stretching exercises. Please note that some of these students have been with me for two years and longer, and they still have pain with only a moderate increase in flexibility. Is there anything that we can do with them or show them so as to alleviate this pain and discomfort? Should they be taking anything—for example, shark cartilage or some other joint building supplement? And will they ever get over this hurdle?

Answer: They should learn the proper alignment of the hips for static and dynamic side stretches. See pages 35, 61, and 112.

Question: Although I come within one foot of a full side split, my range of motion in dynamic stretches (when I swing my leg out to the side) is much worse. Why is this?

Answer: Make sure that you let your pelvis tilt forward (or move buttocks to the rear) when you raise your leg to the side. This action permits raising your leg higher—just as tilting your pelvis forward helps in the side split.

Many people experience quite a bit of discomfort, even pain, in attempting this dynamic stretch. They can only raise each leg to about 45 degrees (and it hurts them when they do that).

Their problem? They try to keep their leg straight, and to raise it straight sideways while attempting to keep their whole body straight too. This is typically the cause of difficulties and hip pain among beginners attempting this leg raise.

To dramatically increase the height of the leg raise to the side, you need to tilt your pelvis forward as you raise your leg sideways. The alignment of hip, thigh, lower leg, and foot in a raising side kick should be the same as shown in a side view of the horse-riding stance (see page 63). To learn its proper form do this: Stand with your feet together, extend your right arm to the side, hand at your hip level, palm down. Slightly bend your right leg in the hip and knee joints. Form your foot correctly (knife foot, *sokuto* in karate, *balnal* in taekwondo) for the side kick (big toe up, rest of toes down, edge of foot horizontal and tensed). Raise the right leg such that you kick your palm with the side of your foot. Start from hip level, and gradually increase the height of leg raises. Make sure that you lean forward and your knee is slightly bent, and that it raises ahead of your foot. Kicking your palm forces you to align your trunk, pelvis, and thigh just right for the greatest range of motion in your hip joints. Note especially the amount and direction of the forward lean in the drawings below.

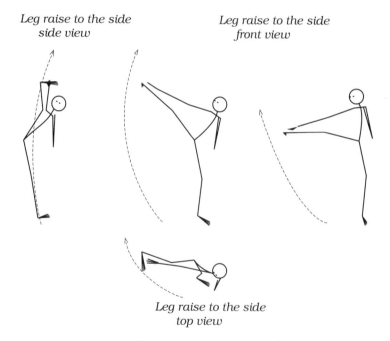

Leg raise to the side
side view

Leg raise to the side
front view

Leg raise to the side
top view

Another purpose of kicking your palm is to keep this dynamic stretch from turning into a ballistic, uncontrolled stretch and to prevent overstretching.

Question: I am into my second week of doing the early morning stretch, *i.e.*, the leg swings. The only problem is that when I swing my leg to the side (and sometimes the front) my back clicks in about the center of my spine. I do not click when I bend my knee when I bring my leg back down. Will I get the same stretch if I bend my knee when bringing my leg down from the swing?

Answer: Yes. I would suggest checking the strength of your back muscles to see if their weakness relative to the psoas causes the clicking.

[Two weeks later the same reader wrote: By the way my back is better. For the side swings I don't think I was leaning forward or twisting my upper body in the direction of the swing enough. Doing that seems to have done the trick.]

Question: I find that any extended use of lateral movement in the hips, such as for the side kick or the roundhouse kick, causes a dull ache in my hips. This is even true when I try to do morning dynamic stretches. It seems my hips interfere more than my muscles. They seem to pop a lot too, when doing the morning dynamic stretch. Do I have any hope to work through this to achieve flexibility for taekwondo kicking? Is there some way to help my hip strength and mobility?

Answer: Make sure that you align your thighs, hips, and trunk as shown on pages 35, 112, and 132 for leg raises to the side (dynamic stretches) and on the video *Power High Kicks with No Warm-Up!* for side and roundhouse kicks. If your hips ache even though you do these movements as shown in this book and on the video, then see an orthopedic surgeon.

Question: When I try to raise my leg to the side my foot turns outward. Is this due to the tightness of the muscles in the leg and hip? How do I get over this?

Answer: Turning of the foot outward during leg raises to the side may be caused by tightness of the muscles that rotate your thigh outward (external rotators of the hip). Try to increase your hips' internal rotation by stretching your external hip rotators. See the stretches on pages 66 and 83.

Question: What is the difference between leg raises or front splits with the front leg straight and bent at the knee?

Answer: The angle between the thighs in a front split and in front raise (kick) is greater, or it is easier to increase it, when the front leg is bent at the knee because your hamstring is relaxed then. Exercise with your front leg straight to better stretch the hamstring.

Hamstrings originate *above* the hip joint and attach *below* the knee joint. Bending your knee relieves the tension of the hamstring and thus permits a greater range of flexion in the hip joint. In a full front split, your pelvis is always tilted to the front in relation to the front thigh no matter what you do with your knees. Tilting of the pelvis is necessary for relaxing the iliofemoral ligament of the hip joint of the rear thigh (see page 109). You can achieve a greater amount of forward tilt when the knee of the front leg is bent because then the hamstring of your front leg is more relaxed.

Question: I can do a front split but when I attempt a side split I get a certain amount of inches off the ground and when I try to slide further into a deeper position I can't because my hips won't let me and the next workout session the outside of my hips are sore and tight. How can I increase the flexibility of my hips so that I may complete the side split?

Answer: Your problem is addressed on pages 61–62 and 111–112 in this book. If you can align the hips and thighs as shown on the Test of Flexibility Potential then all you need to do is to rest until your hips are not sore anymore and then practice your stretches starting from the position shown on page 61. If you cannot perform the test or assume the position shown on page 61 in this book then perhaps the structure of your hip joints (the length and angulation of the neck of your thigh) does not allow sufficient mobility for side split. In that case you better stop trying before you injure your hips.

Question: I practice hamstring stretches lying on my back, but I am a bit confused as to whether it is a good idea to flatten the back or to maintain the curve in the lower back. Can you shed some light on this?

Answer: In such a stretch keeping your back straight or maintaining normal lumbar lordosis stretches mainly the hamstrings. Arching your back (the opposite of lumbar lordosis) will put considerable stretch on the back muscles.

Dynamic Stretches and Morning Stretch

Question: When you describe "leg raises," you refer to a slow, controlled lifting of the leg, not a quick swinging action, correct?

Answer: Controlled, yes, but not very slow. See page 32.

Question: I am 39 years old and I am a relatively new student of taekwondo (4 months). I have been using your book *Stretching Scientifically* with much success. My concern is with my leg raises to the side (dynamic stretches). I am unable to kick my hand, as it seems that my legs are too long (or my arm too short) to do this on the side. I can do so with the front stretches, but when I try with the side I usually only reach my calf at best. I have tried holding something in my hand that "extends" my reach, but I don't always have something available, and this feels awkward. When I have nothing, I usually try to fix a level to attain such as a mark on the wall, to use as a reference point. I don't seem to have any problems, but it seems that my stretches could be moving into ballistic territory without a fixed target. Advice?

Answer: Having a stop, for example, the hand, for your leg raises or kicks, is important only at high velocities of movement. When you do your leg raises slow you do not need any stop.

When you do the raises fast you can try bending the knee of the raising leg more and you can make contact with the lower part of the shin, or use a kicking paddle instead of your hand if your legs are "too long." The higher you raise your leg sideways over your head, the closer you are to kicking your hand.

Question: When I do the leg raises to the back (dynamic stretches), I feel the stretch in the hamstring of my supporting leg, as opposed to the quad of the leg that is being worked. Is this normal?

Answer: Yes. The "weakest link" is the first to respond in any exercise.

Question: If doing dynamic stretches every morning resets the nervous control of muscular length, can't static stretches be done in the morning to achieve the same effect, except for static flexibility rather than dynamic? So then if every morning I did static stretching, I wouldn't need a warm-up to achieve full static flexibility, would I?

Answer: Perhaps, but I do not know. The athletes who use the method of stretching explained in the book *Stretching Scientifically* for a few months can display their maximal static flexibility at any time anyway.

To find out the effect of doing a static stretch in the morning would take an experiment that is not likely to be ever conducted.

Why? Because from the viewpoint of practice-oriented coaches not every question is worthy of research.

You see, doing dynamic stretches in the morning gives an observable increase in athletes' dynamic flexibility later in the day whether or not the athletes do any full ROM (range of motion) static stretches in their morning or evening workouts.

But athletes who do full ROM static stretches invariably do dynamic stretches (or fast movements throughout the full range of motion) too. So finding out what helps them show large ROM in static stretches—whether it is due to dynamic stretches done in the morning, or to static stretches done in the morning, or just an effect of static stretches done during their regular workouts—requires conducting an experiment that could interfere with their training.

Those who achieve full ROM through isometric stretches after a few months of continuing training can display their full range of motion (for example, do a split) anytime—even though initially this did require warming up. This is much like lifting weights—for a beginner establishing a new personal record may require carefully warming up, but with continuous training, after a few months, the same weight may be lifted cold.

What and When

For every rule there is an exception—but you need to know the "why" of the rule and the "why" and "how" of the exception.

Question: When do I do dynamic stretches, when strength exercises, and when isometric stretches?

Answer: Do dynamic stretches at least twice per day, once in the morning and once during a warm-up for your workout.

Do strength training 2–3 times per week, ending with isometric stretches.

Question: What sequence of stretches do I follow since some kicks hurt my back (I have had back surgery)?

Answer: Eliminate stretches that hurt your back.

Question: Do I do the stretch routines after my cardio [endurance workout] or after my weights?

Answer: After both. After a strength workout include isometric stretches in your stretching routine. After an endurance workout do not do isometric stretches but rather static relaxed stretches.

Question: Can I do an early morning stretch after having my breakfast?

Answer: Yes, if you can perform a sufficient number of leg raises with adequate intensity and height without throwing up your breakfast.

Question: Can I do any kinds of stretches (relaxed, for example) after my morning workout?

Answer: Yes, you can do relaxed static stretches after the morning workout. It will not do any harm if you will not do any full power or maximal force movements for a couple of hours afterward.

Question: I jog or run every morning. Will running or jogging after the early morning stretch adversely affect my whole day's flexibility?

Answer: For the running or jogging done after the early morning stretch to adversely affect your flexibility, you would have to considerably fatigue the muscles of your legs.

Question: How long should you rest between sets of dynamic stretches?

Answer: What for? If you need to rest between sets of dynamic stretches you should see a doctor!

Question: While I do not do static stretching to warm up, but rather dynamic (by the by, this has really improved my warm-up time, thanks), I was wondering if it is necessary after the end of a workout (especially if I did isometric stretching) to do relaxed static stretches? Or is it safe to skip them? Are there any real benefits to performing them?

Answer: The benefit of doing isometric and relaxed static stretching is increased passive range of motion and a reduced amount of force needed to hold a stretch—that is, the tension in stretched-out positions. The relaxed stretches permit staying in maximally extended positions longer than the isometric stretches. Doing the relaxed static stretches after isometric stretches may augment these benefits.

If you are not interested in increasing your static flexibility, then do not do static stretches.

Question: How many static stretches should I do in my workout?

Answer: Pick one or two isometric stretches—for example, one for adductors and one for hamstrings—and one or two relaxed stretches for the same muscles. Do as many sets of isometric stretches as you need to reach your current maximum range of motion, but do not force yourself if your muscles are tired and stale. Three to five sets per stretch should be enough. Then, after isometric stretches, you can do relaxed stretches for one or two minutes each.

Question: Is it safe to do six or seven sets of isometric stretches in one workout?

Answer: It should be safe as long as you do not feel pain while exercising. I would not be surprised, though, if you were so sore after this workout that you would have to rest the stretched muscles for a few days. In isometric stretches, as with most strength exercises, it is neither safe nor necessary to exhaust the muscles.

Question: In your opinion, is it better to separate the isometric stretching of the front and side splits (on alternate days, for example)?

Answer: Isometric stretches for both splits can be done in one workout either in the way shown in chapter 7, "Sample Workout Plans," or as is shown on the video *Secrets of Stretching* where after a set of stretches leading to the side split I stand in a deep lunge and tense the legs. You may also work on one of the splits until you reach your desired ROM. It all depends on the individual.

To make the right decision you need to pay attention to your body and not disregard its warnings. You also need to be in good shape. Isometric stretches require normal strength, which in the case of legs means being able to comfortably do at least 10 squats with a barbell of a weight equal to your body weight. Even with normal strength you need to be well rested to attempt isometric stretches. By the way, proper strength preparation (resulting in greater than the above described minimum strength) before learning the techniques of kicking prevents knee problems and other joint problems too.

Question: The mornings are the best time of the day for my karate workouts. Can I do isometric stretches at the end of those morning karate workouts or do I have to do isometric stretches in the evening?

Answer: It depends on your objective. If having great dynamic flexibility without a warm-up during the day is not your objective, then you can do isometrics in the morning. If you want to be flexible during the remainder of the day after your morning karate workout, you can postpone isometrics as well as other strenuous strength exercises until late afternoon or evening. Just make sure that you warm up well. You always have to monitor your progress; if your strength and flexibility keep improving while you do isometrics in the morning workouts, then it is fine to do them then.

Question: I know that you have recommended many times not to do static stretches before dynamic martial art practices [see pages 21, 22, and 122 for a detailed explanation]. Unfortunately, most martial arts schools that I have seen do static stretches as part of their warm-up, mine included. For numerous reasons, I do not want to leave the school, so I have adapted a "system" to get around this problem and would appreciate your comments. First, I arrive at class early, and I spend about 5–10 minutes warming up, and then I do my dynamic leg stretches. I then go out to class, which usually starts with some running in place or around the dojang, push-ups, sit-ups, and then some static stretching. When this part comes, I simply get into the positions, but I don't really push the stretch at all. Sometimes I will feel a very minor stretch in some of the positions, but that is all. Is this an effective way to get around the stretching issue, or are there problems even with this "light" stretching?

Answer: Yes, it is an effective way of dealing with an ignorant instructor. Just standing in a position and pretending to stretch will do you no harm. It is not what the thing is called—for instance, a static stretch—but what it does that matters. If you stretch not at all or very little, then you will not weaken your muscles.

Be very cautious when you actually stretch statically at the end of the workout, or any time you assume a "stretching" position, because some morons have been known to approach a stretching athlete and push him or her into a greater stretch.

Question: Do static stretches have to be part of a workout, or can I do them by themselves?

Answer: It is better to do them at the end of the workout when your muscles are well warmed up. This applies particularly to isometric stretches. You can do relaxed stretches by themselves, when you have already cooled down from a workout, but do them slowly so you do not hurt unprepared muscles. Such stretching will be more difficult and less effective than stretching when you are warmed up.

Question: Since reading your book and viewing the video *Secrets of Stretching*, I have decided to redo my workout routines. Even though I want to develop a workout that will improve my karate skills and flexibility, I also want to maintain and even improve my muscle mass in my upper body.

Here is what I have come up with:
Days 1, 2, 3, 5, and 6: Dynamic Stretching A.M. & P.M.
Day 1 & 6: Technical/Speed (techniques & kicking drills, sparring)
Day 2 & 5: Strength. I have listed the exercises in the order I do them. [The list of resistance exercises shows isolation exercises before complex movements (leg extensions and leg curls before squats and deadlifts), exercises for stabilizing muscles before the prime movers (deadlifts before hip adductors and hip flexor exercises, abdomen exercises before back extensions).]
Day 3: Aerobics (jump rope, running/sprints, relaxed stretching)
Day 4: Off

What do you think?

Answer: Both the video *Secrets of Stretching* and the book *Stretching Scientifically* (pages 52 and 53) explain how to schedule workouts, but you managed to miss it. Your Technical or Speed workout must precede your Strength or Endurance workout, a Strength workout must precede any Endurance workout, which is followed by a day of complete rest or active rest (easy, fun activity). Do not do a Technical or Speed workout on the day immediately following either an exhausting Strength or an exhausting Endurance workout, and do not do a Strength workout before fully recovering after an exhausting Endurance workout because such sequences of efforts lead to overtraining.

In single workouts do not work on endurance before any other ability with the exception of static passive flexibility, which is developed by relaxed stretches. Study *Science of Sports Training* for an in-depth explanation of why the same exercises give different results depending on their sequence in a workout and in the weekly sequence of workouts.

Regarding your strength exercises, I suggest that, instead of leg curls and extensions, you do more squats and deadlifts since they are better for your knees. By doing the deadlifts before adductor exercises, and abdomen crunches before back extensions, you break the rule of never fatiguing the stabilizers—in this instance, your back, which stabilizes your legs, or abdomen muscles, which stabilize your back—before the prime movers.

Question: The best time for me to do my isometric stretches and strengthening exercises is late at night, around 23:30 or midnight. Will this have any effect on my flexibility gains or does it matter?

Answer: Late night is not the best time for working out but if the exercise does not interfere with your sleeping well, then perhaps it is fine for you.

The importance of getting enough of high quality sleep for making progress is explained in the new edition of *Science of Sports Training*. In that book you will also find information on the best times during the day for developing different abilities and skills.

Generally it is better to have a few hours between the end of the workout and going to bed to "walk off" the fatigue, tension, and excitement of the workout. You may want to try doing your strengthening and stretching exercises in several short sessions, each dedicated to one body part, during the day rather than in one long session late at night. For example, squats and isometric stretches in the first session, deadlifts and relaxed stretches in the second session, or deadlifts alone in the second session, and relaxed stretches in the third, final session.

Stretching in Workouts for Various Sports

Athletes who ask me what stretches they should do astound me. Don't they practice their sport and know their moves? Don't they feel which of their movements are restricted by tight muscles? A typical question goes: I have your book *Stretching Scientifically;* however, I was hoping for something geared solely for a ___ [name of any sport here]. Do you have anything on stretching that is designed for ___? My answer: *Stretching Scientifically* shows stretches for most muscle groups and so anyone can find in it stretches to suit any sport or individual need. Nevertheless, readers keep asking, so here are some specifics.

Question: Is it recommendable to do relaxed (static passive) stretches during a bodybuilding workout, e.g., stretching the pectoralis muscles between two sets of bench presses?

Answer: It depends on the amount of resistance in your lifts and on how strenuously you stretch. The greater the resistance the more dangerous it is to do strenuous static stretches between sets. Maximal force production is impaired for several minutes after strenuous static stretching. Your own lifting experience should tell you that. Research confirms it too (Kokkonen et al. 1998).

Maximal force production in purely concentric (from a standstill) bench press, one of the events of powerlifting, is positively related to the stiffness of prime movers (Wilson et al. 1994), so flexibility training could affect it adversely.

Question: I lift weights and have boxing practice in a day. Which one—lifting or boxing—should I use dynamic and isometric stretches before and after?

Answer: Dynamic stretches in warm-ups for either workout, isometric stretches after lifting. Boxing practice as a rule (with very few exceptions) should precede lifting, and the reasons why are explained in the second edition of *Science of Sports Training*.

Question: I want to know if your methods will help increase my flexibility in regard to dance (ballet and jazz). For example, most technical dance kicks require an upright posture with a turned out straight leg from the hip with the pelvis tilted forward. Would following your method be appropriate for the kind of body alignments I need to achieve or would they work against my goals?

Answer: The method of stretching described in *Stretching Scientifically* affects primarily the neural control of muscles and, in the case of isometric stretching, also strengthens muscles in extended positions. It works regardless of the form of your movements as long as the movements themselves are not injurious.

Question: I have been using your stretching techniques for years (off and on since 1989) and have had good results with them. What I am now interested in is stretching methods specifically to enhance the golf swing, i.e., to improve the shoulder turn and increase speed and strength throughout the swing.

Answer: During your golf swing practice you feel which muscle groups limit your mobility and in which positions. Find in this book the stretches that give you a similar feeling, or using the principles of stretching you know from the book, design stretches to suit your need.

Question: Would doing all stretches for all the body parts be too much flexibility training for karate?

Answer: I think it would be too much for any sport and for anybody's muscles.

Question: How should I introduce this method into my martial arts workout?

Answer: Do dynamic stretches at the beginning of your workout, after the aerobic part of the warm-up. Then do your techniques or sparring. At the end of the workout, do your strength or conditioning exercises, then do isometric stretches and follow them with relaxed stretches. If you do your strength exercises in a separate workout, then do dynamic stretches in the warm-up, and isometric stretches at the end of that workout. Do relaxed stretches in the cool-down of any workout, either after isometric stretches or instead of them. I do not recommend doing isometric stretches every day. Two to four times per week, depending on the reaction of your muscles, is enough.

Question: I do martial arts and, two to three times a week, after each gym workout with weights, I run for cardiovascular conditioning. This being the case, when should I incorporate isometric, and relaxed stretches, after lifting and before running, or at the end after both? (This first session I did, I stretched after the run, as my final exercise, and did not seem to experience anything untoward.) I've always thought stretching is to be done at the very end, to return muscles to their original relaxed length after training.

Answer: First, an endurance run (even only 20 minutes long) after a strength training workout, reduces gains in strength. This is because of the conflicting demands that strength work and aerobic endurance work put on the body in general and on the muscle fibers in particular. This issue is explained in several standard texts on exercise physiology. This conflict is most pronounced if you use very heavy resistance, such as when attempting to increase maximal strength, and less pronounced when you are using moderate resistance in a high number of reps, such as when working on muscular endurance.

Usually athletes do their strength workouts on different days than aerobic endurance workouts, with a period of rest between these workouts such that fatigue from one kind of work does not impair the ability to perform the other. The preferred arrangement is with aerobic endurance done right after the technical or speed workout and maximal strength work done in a separate workout on a different day—but it all depends on the current priorities and on your speed of recovery, which depends on how much you run and lift. Dedicating a separate workout to strength is usually done when developing maximal strength is the priority. In this event, work on the aerobic endurance is reduced so fatigue from it does not interfere with strength workouts and the strength workout is the first or second (after technique) in the weekly schedule.

All this notwithstanding, if your schedule works for you, then stick to it—as long as you are satisfied with your progress.

Second, isometric stretches are strength exercises so they may lose some effectiveness (as far as increasing strength in the stretched positions) if done after an endurance run. I think it is best to do them at the end of a strength workout, after other strength exercises. If you want to do isometric stretches together with your running, then it may be better to do them before the run, and relaxed stretches after the run.

Question: What stretches do you recommend doing before and after running?

Answer: Before long-distance running you can forgo stretching and then do all your stretches after running in the sequence given on pages 23 and 24. For middle distances and sprints I suggest the following warm-up and stretches: light jogging plus arm circles and arm swings, light jogging plus kick heels to buttocks, march with heel to toe raises, leg raises to the front, leg raises to the back, leg swings front to back while standing on one leg. After the run do either isometric or relaxed stretches—one for the calves, then one for the hamstrings, and one for hip flexors. If you are not very fatigued after your run, you can also do dynamic stretches for legs before the relaxed stretches.

If some of your muscles are so tight before any run that you think you need to stretch them just to run well—then I think you should see a doctor and not be running.

Question: Are you aware of any long-term adverse effects of running or strength training on flexibility?

Answer: No, running or strength training have no adverse effect on flexibility provided you train rationally, do exercises in the correct sequence, and provide adequate rest to your body.

Question: I skate. What stretches would you suggest for in-line skating?

Answer: Before putting the skates on do leg raises to the front, back, and sides. With the skates on get a hold on some support (a bench or rail), and do squats and deep lunges to stretch the muscles that limit your range of motion. Gradually increase range of motion by either extending legs further back or lowering hips more. After skating do either isometric or relaxed stretches—one for the hip flexors that also stretches the shins (see page 67 and page 85), then one for your hamstrings, and finally one for your inner thigh muscles.

Question: How should skiers warm-up and stretch?

Answer: Stretches for cross-country skiers: First warm-up with walking and then running with some side-to-side agility movements to warm up ankles and knees. Then do dynamic stretches such as leg raises before putting the skis on. After putting the skis on, do turns and twists in one spot, and then get into a deep lunge position and switch legs sliding them back and forth. Do not get tired doing this before the run. After the run you can do it until your legs are tired.

Stretches for downhill skiers: First warm-up with walking and then running with some agility movements (side to side hops or jumps). Then do dynamic stretches such as leg raises before putting the boots on, then with boots and skis on do turns and twists in one spot. After skiing, while still on the skis, go down on a very gentle slope spreading legs wide and then bringing them together several times, which is similar to isometric stretches.

Question: What would be proper warm-up and stretches for swimmers?

Answer: Warm-up and stretches for swimmers: arm circles and swings first out of water then in the water (so a part of the movement is done against resistance). After swimming: take a towel or a rope or a stick and do isometric or relaxed stretches for the arms. Then do isometric or relaxed stretches—one for hip flexors and quads, then one for hamstrings or one for both lower back and hamstrings, and one abdomen and hip flexors stretch.

Question: Would doing weightlifting and all kinds of stretches in a workout be too much for one's muscles?

Answer: This depends on the person and the selection of exercises (including stretches). If you do not feel sore after such workouts then they are probably okay.

Flexibility and Other Athletic Abilities

Question: Sometimes when I try to do isometric stretching to my maximum reach, my leg starts to shake. Do you have any idea why that might happen?

Answer: Perhaps the shaking is caused by impaired inter - and intramuscular coordination due to fatigue. If so, then it might be remedied by improved muscular strength or muscular endurance.

Question: How many times per week should one do isometric stretches? Is it the same as with lifting weights, in which case each body part is exercised 2 or 3 times per week?

Answer: Both isometrics and lifting weights are strength exercises. They both should be done during the same workout (strength workout). More information on this and on related subjects is in the book *Science of Sports Training.*

Question: I am the only person at my club who lifts weights, so your methods are really convenient for me, but can the others expect to attain maximum flexibility without entering the gym?

Answer: Strength training is necessary for martial arts and it helps with developing flexibility but it does not have to be done with iron weights. Bodyweight exercises and exercises with a partner— for example, during and at the end of a typical martial arts workout—can be done instead of standard exercises with weights.

Question: I want to increase my vertical jump and maximize my flexibility. My coaches tell me I have to stretch my hamstrings, calf muscles and Achilles tendon to reach peak jumping ability. Is it true?

Answer: I do not think that improved flexibility of the legs will be of any help in jumping up if you have normal range of motion in the hips, knees, and ankles.

If you want to know how to combine exercises developing strength, jumping ability, flexibility, and other abilities in your workouts for optimum results, read *Explosive Power and Jumping Ability for All Sports.*

Question: Do you believe that larger muscles make you less flexible than smaller ones?

Answer: If you define flexibility as a passive range of extension (how far can you extend your joints passively), then no—larger muscles do not make you less flexible. If you define flexibility as a passive range of flexion (how much can you flex your joints passively), then yes—larger muscles can make you less flexible than smaller ones.

Question: Can relaxed stretching exercises prevent muscles from becoming bulky or big?

Answer: No.

Question: How do my isometric stretches change once I am able to lift myself up from the floor while in a split?

Answer: If you want to further increase the strength of your hamstrings and adductors, you can try to increase their tension by holding weights in your hands, or put a weighted belt on, or press or pull against some immovable object.

Question: To increase resistance and thus the tension of my muscles in a split, I hold a long stick and press it against the ceiling while trying to lift myself from the split. What do you think about such a way of increasing resistance?

Answer: Your idea of using a long stick that touches the ceiling to add resistance has an advantage over my method of holding weights—it allows you to apply resistance at precise angles and in moments that you choose. It also seems safer than holding weights because you can apply tension gradually and release it faster than you can throw down the dumbbells. The drawback, comparing the use of the stick to dumbbells, is that you do not know precisely how much resistance you apply.

Question: You say that in an attempt to develop exceptional strength and flexibility one should combine isometric stretches with dynamic strength exercises such as lifting weights. If lifting weights, what exercises do you recommend?

Answer: Squats, lunges, step-ups, deadlifts, good mornings.

Question: I would like to know how you feel about free weights for someone who plays tennis and is studying aikido [or trains for any two or more sports]. Do you recommend using free weights as a supplementary form of exercise for these athletic endeavors, or do you feel that doing all three forms of stretching is sufficient? If you do believe in using free weights, what routine would you recommend for the above sports?

Answer: Resistance exercises are necessary in sports training, even if the particular sport seems to require little strength, as a means of injury prevention and of preparing the body for intensive technical workouts. No stretches can replace free weights as a means of graduated resistance training. I cannot give you any "routine" for use of free weights because the choice of exercises depends on too many constantly changing factors for any routine to be useful and I cannot teach you the methodology of sports training in a few sentences. Instead, I recommend the video *Secrets of Stretching*, which covers the principles of general athletic conditioning, strength, and flexibility training, or the book *Science of Sports Training*.

Question: Yesterday I did a workout with a lot of kicking and today my hamstrings are sore. Is this due to my muscles not being strong enough? Or not flexible enough? What should I do to stop my hamstrings from getting sore? They do not get sore after lifting weights—only after kicking.

Answer: Muscle soreness is a sign that the structural strength of muscles is not comfortably above the demand put on these muscles. Kick less and lift more. Make sure that you move through the full range of motion and gradually add more weight in such exercises as squats, good mornings, and stiff-legged deadlifts. Increase the number of kicks in your workouts *gradually.*

Question: Why do you advise doing long sets of exercises with low resistance as a preparation for low-repetition and high-resistance strength exercises and isometric stretches?

Answer: My recommendations increase the structural strength of the muscles so they are less likely to be excessively damaged by strenuous exercises. (Excessive muscle damage announces itself as delayed-onset muscle soreness, or a muscle strain, even a complete muscle rupture.) The structural strength of a muscle is determined by the strength and cross-sectional area of the slow-twitch muscle fibers and by the strength of the connective tissue within the muscle. Slow-twitch muscle fibers have relatively greater structural strength than fast-twitch fibers, especially the fast-twitch fibers with low oxidative capacities (Fridén and Lieber 1992; Lieber and Fridén 2000). It takes more force to stretch, and ultimately to rupture, the slow-twitch fibers than the fast-twitch fibers. This is because the slow-twitch fibers are smaller than the fast-twitch fibers and have a greater ratio of cellular scaffolding to the contractile elements (which are built of long, thin proteins that are easy to tear).

Endurance training, that is, doing many repetitions per set against low resistance, increases the structural strength of slow-twitch muscle fibers (Gleim and McHugh 1997). Such training also increases the structural strength of the connective tissue within the muscle, probably through the anabolic action of hormones that are delivered to the muscle with the increased blood flow (Tipton et al. 1975). The connective tissue damage is considered another one of the causes of delayed-onset muscle soreness (McArdle, Katch, and Katch 1996).

Question: Don't you reduce the flexibility of your legs when you do kicking endurance training for your legs?

Answer: Not if you maintain your flexibility with an increased amount of stretching—as much as it takes to reach your normal range of motion in the cool-down stretches after the workout and next day in the dynamic stretches of the morning stretch.

Question: I know you recommend deep and heavy squats for leg strength. I train at home and don't have a spotter; nor do I have time to go to a gym. I'm a kickboxer and would like to improve my leg strength for use in my sport, and I was wondering what alternative to very heavy squats I might use, seeing as how it's not feasible to squat heavy without a spotter. Are there other exercises I could do that would produce a similar level of leg strength?

Answer: Squats and deadlifts are the easiest lifts to self-spot. If you need a spotter for a squat, then you are lifting too much—especially in that you are a kickboxer and not a powerlifter. A person who trains progressing gradually can self-spot squats with the help of a rack or, in emergency, can easily dump the bar weighing more than one's body weight.

Question: I don't have any weights to do squats or deadlifts. Can I substitute doing a high number of repetitions of weight-free squats (3 sets of 100 repetitions)?

Answer: Weight-free squats may strengthen your whole body, but mainly your thighs. The weight-free squats will have little effect on the muscles of your lower back which are best strengthened with deadlift-like movements against considerable resistance.

Question: When one does dynamic strength exercises for the groin and hamstrings in preparation for isometric stretches, is it better (or necessary) to do the exercises using the full range of motion? For example, regular hamstring curls use a very limited range of motion, whereas stiff-legged deadlifts work the muscle in a stretched position.

Answer: Generally, yes, do the strength exercises in the full range of motion. You may consider doing heavy deadlifts *after* all your isometric stretches for hips. Isometric stretches leading to the side split and the front split involve strong tensions of psoas muscles that attach to the front of the lumbar spine. Back erectors are fatigued by doing stabilizing work during heavy deadlifts, back extensions, or "good mornings" and so may spasm during isometric stretches for the splits.

Question: I dare not do normal squats with a barbell because my whole hip and inner thigh areas tighten up for around ten days, despite stretching in the morning, before and after training. If I just do hack squats I can wake up in the morning and do a full front and side split. Doing hack squats alone avoids targeting the inner thigh muscles (this is why I am very flexible, without touching the inner thighs). If I don't touch any weights I drop into splits most times of the day.

Answer: The most likely cause of this excessive soreness and tightness after strength exercises is that you are not starting with sufficiently low weights to match the weakness of your muscles and then you are not progressing gradually enough so as not to overwork them. Every time you feel tightness, you become alarmed and abandon the exercise that exposed your weakness, and then wonder why you stay weak in that area. For the short-time satisfaction of being able to do splits without warm-up now, you forsake any further development of both strength and flexibility.

Question: If a lack of strength in the adductor muscles prevents doing a side split, does this suggest that a junior high cheerleader who does splits easily has typically stronger adductors than, for example, an Olympic decathlete who cannot?

Answer: The lack of strength in the adductors of the thigh prevents achieving and performing on demand a side split if you are using isometric stretches.

Yes, typically a little girl who can slide down into a split and then can raise herself up from that split can have thigh adductors stronger (in relation to her body weight) at the angles and extensions occurring in the split than a decathlete who can't, even though his absolute muscular strength may be greater. For explanation of the difference between relative muscular strength and absolute muscular strength see *Science of Sports Training*.

Question: A few months ago, I began training to do the Olympic lifts (snatch and clean and jerk). I am so stiff that I can't receive the bar correctly in the clean. The main problem seems to be my inability to flex my hips fully while keeping my lower back extended. This prevents me from keeping my torso upright, and the bar falls forward off my shoulders. Two lesser but still significant problems are getting my elbows high enough; and flexing my ankles far enough in the low squat so as to remain balanced front to back without leaning forward. The net effect of these problems is that I simply can't do a correct clean. Can you suggest any exercises or warm-ups to help with these problems?

Answer: Your problems can be remedied by doing lots of deep and wide squats without a barbell and with a barbell in both front squat and back squat positions. For dynamic flexibility do these squats fast with light weights and for static flexibility do them slow but with heavier weights.

You might benefit from reading up on an analysis of the lifts. Some of the better books on this subject are available from Iron-Mind (P.O. Box 1228, Nevada City, CA 95959, phone 530-265-6725).

Question: I had never done much in the way of weight training before, and late last year I suffered a shoulder injury. I was told that I was probably not stretching my shoulders properly before and after weight training. (I was having most problems with the incline bench press.)

Having studied your video on kicking I am uncertain that the stretching methods I have been shown are the most effective. These are static stretches resisting against a wall. Your "law of specificity" makes me wonder if there is a better way. Can you enlighten me?

Answer: I never do any form of static stretching prior to weight lifting or any resistance exercises. Static stretches temporarily weaken and predispose to injury the stretched muscles. Static stretches are to be done after and not before resistance exercises but I am not aware of any detrimental effect of not stretching the shoulders after the resistance exercises. After all, if the resistance exercises are done within normal range of motion, they will not reduce it.

Your problem may have more to do with doing too much too soon, improper form of movements, or improper balance of exercises.

Question: You don't like hanging back stretches because of possible ligament stretching, but you recommend stiff-leg deadlifts. So, do you recommend only bending over to a certain extent when deadlifting, i.e., the weight lowered only to knee or midcalf?

Answer: When done correctly, the deadlift does not stretch lower back ligaments nor even the lower back muscles. Information on how to do a deadlift is in article 21 of my column on training ("Advanced Strength Exercises for Lower Back—Your Best Insurance against Back Pain" posted at http://www.stadion.com/column.html) and in the Summer 1996 issue of *Stadion News* downloadable from our site.

Question: I have been doing taekwondo for seven years now and the stretching done in class (far too quick and not in the correct sequence that you recommend) has never really improved my flexibility. I find that if I skip training in any form for about a week or two I am *more* flexible but then get sore later after resuming my taekwondo workout. Even when following your guide, after a taekwondo session I am too sore and stiff (in my hamstrings) to work out daily by your method. What is the cause of my soreness and lack of progress in flexibility?

Answer: There are two possible causes of your lack of progress in flexibility development:

1. The taekwondo workouts are run by a possibly good fighter but a lousy coach. (You said that exercises are not done in the correct sequence.)

2. Your muscles are too weak for these workouts. Soreness after a workout indicates it.

My advice is to stop attending taekwondo workouts and gradually bring your flexibility, strength, and endurance to such a level that after a few month you can safely return to taekwondo.

Your training has to be systematic, with gradually increasing workloads. Follow the advice from this book or the video *Secrets of Stretching*.

Question: How many times a week should I do strength exercises before I perform the isometric stretches?

Answer: The most accurate answer is: As many times as it takes to get strong enough for the isometric stretches.

Strength training is not treated in depth in *Stretching Scientifically* because it is a guide to flexibility training for athletes—people already familiar with strength training. This book is for athletes who want to update their knowledge of flexibility training and maximize its effectiveness. For strength training information, see either chapter 6, "Strength," of the book *Science of Sports Training* or the book *Explosive Power and Jumping Ability for All Sports*. All you need to know about strength training as it relates to isometric stretches is in chapter 5, pages 49–53 of *Stretching Scientifically*.

A simple rule for those new to strength training: Typically, strength exercises for a given muscle group are done two or three times per week. How often you should do strength exercises depends on your reaction to them. If your muscles are sore the next day after every strength workout, even if you make some progress, it means that you exercise too often or too much. If you do not get muscle soreness but make poor progress, it may mean that you should either exercise more often or increase the number of repetitions or the resistance.

Question: You recommend using dynamic strength exercises until the muscles are ready for isometric stretches. I do two sets of 30 repetitions for each muscle group (groin, hamstrings) three times every two weeks. Is this often enough? I get sore if I do the exercises any more frequently than that. Which is better: A hard workout once a week, or a lighter workout twice a week?

Answer: Slow but steady is better.

Question: When I stretch out for a taekwondo class, I find that for the next two days I am sore and stiff in groin muscles. From your book, I read that this is a sign that those muscles are too weak. This is the case where long sets of high reps to the point of burn are used, correct?

Answer: Perhaps they are too weak, or perhaps you do too much. Long sets of movements at full range of motion will help if the muscles are too weak, but not if you already do too much.

Question: Here is my general workout week. Dynamic stretch every morning and evening. I do no isometric stretches yet as I fear that my muscles and tendons are unprepared for them. I am anxious to begin to help my gross inflexibility problems.

Monday, Wednesday, Friday: Weight training, kicking drills, 1–2 mile run. Tuesday, Thursday: Taekwondo class. Saturday: Light endurance workout. Sunday: Off

Answer: Doing weight training prior to kicking drills as well as weight training for lower body and running on the same day are strange practices. In your case, because you run so little, running on the same day as lifting weights may have no adverse effect on your strength. But if you are serious about your fighting form, why do you run so little? Proper arrangements of workouts are explained in the book *Science of Sports Training.*

Question: I'm 45 and getting back into taekwondo after a 20-year layoff (red belt then). I'm in good shape, but even 20 years ago my flexibility wasn't that great. My goal of course is to do the side split. What do you think of my workouts?

My workout week: morning warm-up, then 1–2 sets leg raises all three directions, some kicking practice, 2 wall squats (lean back against wall, lower down and hold for 60 seconds). Then relaxed static stretches in this order: front of the thigh stretch, inner thigh or butterfly stretch (PNF and relax on this one), lower back stretch, calf and hamstring stretch (PNF and relax style on this also). Then I try doing a side split. Some light jogging and I'm on my way to work as a mailman.

During breaks at work I stretch arms and shoulders, do 2 wall squats leaning against my truck for 60 seconds each, then I do 2 sets of lower back and hamstring stretches. I also do 2 sets of leg stretches, each about 40 sec. After I get home, eat, and shower I do at least one set of 12 dynamic leg raises all three directions. Twice a week I have taekwondo class (usually Monday and Thursday), Wednesday I do Tae-Bo aerobics class. Friday, Saturday, and Sunday are light workout days, no classes but same routine otherwise. I don't work on Sunday and on one other day, it rotates. On my light days I try and squeeze in what I need to know for taekwondo besides kicking, forms, and self-defense.

Answer: I think you do too much. You work out every day of the week as if you did not know that rest is an integral and necessary part of training. A morning stretch should consist of dynamic stretches, perhaps one or two relaxed stretches for some particularly inflexible muscle group, but no isometric or PNF stretches—especially before long physical efforts.

You do too many isometric stretches for too many muscle groups—five muscle groups just in the morning. One isometric stretch per one muscle group, up to three muscle groups stretched per workout is plenty. Change the stretch for a more effective one once it no longer increases range of motion. To reach your goal of a side split, you have to do exercises that are specifically designed for reaching it. You also have to observe your reaction to these exercises and adjust your training accordingly.

Question: You say that bicycling is bad for flexibility of lower limbs. Having been an avid cyclist, I believe you! And you suggest that running is a better alternative for cardiovascular conditioning. True, compared to biking, the range of motion is much greater, but wouldn't using your full range of motion while running introduce a "braking" effect as your front knee would be significantly in front of your center of gravity, in turn causing harmful stress to the knee?

Also, what other cardiovascular activities do you think are not detrimental to flexibility? I can't think of any that use the full range of motion of all the body parts involved.

Answer: My answer to your first question (on the braking effect): No. To see why, view the slow-motion run on the video *Secrets of Stretching*. To have this problem a person would have to be pathologically discoordinated.

Answer to your second question: The activities do not have to use the full range of motion of involved joints—it is enough that the muscles that cross these joints are at or close to their resting length. So, for example, jumping rope does not reduce the range of motion in hip joints, unlike cycling, where most muscles that cross the hip joint work continuously while considerably shortened. Examples of exercises, other than running and rope jumping, that are not detrimental to flexibility are shadow boxing, running up stairs, and cross-country skiing.

Running on skis, whether on the snow or using a Nordic Track or other ski machine, permits full extensions in hip and knee joints, so it does not have the same effect on flexibility as biking.

Age and Stretching

Question: I've seen your ads on learning to do splits after 50, but I'm a bit skeptical. After all, George Dillman [who demonstrates a side split suspended between two chairs, which he achieved at age 50] has been doing martial arts for a long time. I've only been at it 1 year and am over 50. How will your system overcome my lack of flexibility?

Answer: Our method of stretching depends on making your muscles stronger in stretched out positions. It means that you can improve your flexibility as long as you as you can increase your muscular strength. So, if you can make progress lifting more and more weights or overcoming more resistance in any strength exercises, you can stretch more too. To see if your bone structure or ligaments are not going to limit your ability to do splits try our simple Tests of Flexibility Potential shown on pages 108–110.

Question: I am 15 years old and I am anxious to start isometrics as I know that isometric stretches are the quickest way to achieving splits. I have been very inflexible most of my life and I am starting martial arts (taekwondo). I want to know, from a physiological standpoint, why I can't do isometrics. I haven't grown significantly in quite a while. Does this mean I'm ready for more intense training?

Answer: Maybe you can do isometrics and maybe you cannot. It depends on your skeleton's maturity (whether you have finished growing or not) and your physician should be able to tell you one way or the other. My general recommendation is that young people whose bones are still growing do not do isometric stretches, and it's based on the advice from world-renowned authorities (see *Children and Sports Training* and *Science of Sports Training*).

It is recommended that fifteen- and sixteen-year-olds lift weights no heavier than 100% of their body weight. (The rationale is given in *Science of Sports Training*.) For a normal adolescent lifting 100%

of his or her body weight in common lifts such as the squat, deadlift, or bench press requires much less than the maximal muscular contraction, but in isometric stretches muscles are tensed up to the maximal voluntary contraction. That would exceed the magnitude of tension that is considered safe for an immature skeleton.

Because your sport requires kicking and not doing gymnastic splits, I recommend that you concentrate on dynamic stretches as the main means of developing flexibility and do some relaxed static stretches at the end of a cool-down after your workouts.

Question: What should I focus on with the young students— more strengthening, or should I still be focusing on stretching?

Answer: That depends on how young the students are. With little children do mainly dynamic stretches. With older children you can add static relaxed stretches, with young people past puberty you can do all kinds of stretching as long as they are strong enough. Information on strength training for children and youth is in the book *Children and Sports Training: How Your Future Champions Should Exercise to Be Healthy, Fit, and Happy.*

Gender and Stretching

Question: I've seen your ad. How come there are no pictures of women doing the chair (or any) splits?

Answer: Because no woman took the trouble of sending a photo of her side split between chairs. You can be the first.

But seriously—it appears that in martial arts there are even fewer women who undertake serious training than the small number of men who do. In other sports, such as gymnastics, the situation is different and many women gymnasts display such splits easily. This may have to do with the lesser quality of the majority of instructors in martial arts as compared to instructors of gymnastics as well as with the athletes' selection process. Women gymnasts who are rationally trained by well-educated coaches have no need to study my book or video and so do not send testimonials.

Question: Is it true that females are generally more flexible than males?

Answer: It is true only if comparing, for example, hip flexibility of the sexes in the general population, but it is not true for individuals and not necessarily true for other joints. Don't you know men who are more flexible (in all major joints) than many women?

Females all over the world tend to have a greater range of motion in the hip joint and in the elbow (Alter 1996). But results of studies of differences in flexibility done in different countries may vary for other joints. For example, a study done in the U.S.A. by R. E. Koslow (1987) shows that 17- and 21-year-old women have greater range of motion than 17- and 21-year-old men in the shoulder, while a study done in Italy by F. Repice et al. (1982) shows the opposite.

From observation of gymnasts—athletes who are both selected for flexibility and work a lot on flexibility—you can see that women gymnasts *tend* to be more flexible than men of the same skill level. It has to do with differences in the bone structure and perhaps with women gymnasts having more compliant ligaments and usually less muscle mass around all joints than men gymnasts.

Question: Is women's ability to kick high much better than men's?

Answer: If you refer to high martial arts' kicks—delivering hard impact when kicking high—then, based on my observations, I would say no. If you mean dance-like kicks, then women show greater range of motion than men.

Sounds in and around Joints

Questions (from more than one person)

1. I have been doing one of the stretching routines from the book for the past week and have noticed a 10% increase in my flexibility. However, I have noticed that my hips click more than they used to. It doesn't hurt but it does click. Is this a sign that the hip joint is loosening up or do you think I am doing something incorrect in the stretching method?

2. Sometimes when I am stretching, I hear a popping noise in my hip area. After the noise, I seem to be able to stretch a little further. I was just wondering what the popping noise is?

3. Just recently my hip has been popping a lot. At times I have to make it pop in order to feel better. It also sometimes pops just by me

walking. Also my knee does the same thing. What's wrong and should I see a doctor?

4. I am very flexible and fit. However, for the past month or so I have noticed that when I do straight leg front raises or what we call 'axe kicks,' while my foot is coming back down I will feel and hear a popping in my hip joints. What is this from and what should I do about it?

Answer: The nature of noises in the joints is best determined by a competent physician.

Increased flexibility (range of motion) may cause greater frequency of joint clicking or popping, resulting from an enhanced leverage of the joint's bones.

Painless clicking or cracking in the joints themselves is harmless, especially if followed by the feeling of release of tension and by increased mobility. It usually happens when a joint is pulled or bent into a greater range of motion than usual.

There is a negative pressure in the joints. It keeps joint surfaces fitting closely. Joint surfaces normally do not touch each other. A thin layer of synovial fluid between joint cartilages protects them from rubbing against each other and there is gas (of a composition similar to air) dissolved in this fluid.

The cracking sound is caused by this gas dissolving out of the synovial fluid and forming a bubble between joint surfaces when the bones are pulled apart far enough. After several minutes the gas redissolves into the fluid (Alter 1996). Popping or cracking of joints is not harmful per se but may be a sign of joint tightness caused by overly or unevenly tensed muscles—from an improper strength training or a neurological dysfunction.

Popping or snapping outside of the joint cavity may be caused by a ligament or a tendon catching on and then slipping over a bony prominence or by degenerative changes in the joint.

Some noises may be caused by tight muscles. For example, clicking or snapping outside of the hip joint (on the outside of the pelvis) may be caused by a tight iliotibial band and may be relieved by stretches of the hip abductors (gluteus medius, gluteus minimus, tensor fasciae latae, piriformis). Clicking or snapping to the inside of the hip joint (front of the pelvis) may be caused by a tight psoas.

Muscles can become tight as a result of too much effort or too frequent exercise and not enough rest.

Another cause of sounds in a joint is osteoarthritis. When joint surfaces are diseased and the cartilage is eaten away, the ligaments and tendons crossing the joint get slack. Their slack lets them move in and out of their grooves, making popping sounds.

Loose bodies in a joint, making creaking noises particularly in the knee and hip joints, can be a result of chondromalacia (softening of the articular surfaces). This type of degeneration is accompanied by inflammation, pain, and swelling.

Kneecaps may "pop" when they snap in and out of alignment with the thigh bone as knees are bent and straightened. This may be caused by weak quadriceps. Check with a doctor if the knees hurt, swell, or get sore after working out or after walking up or down the stairs.

Clicking in the hip when extending the hip joint (as when dropping the leg after an axe kick) and adducting the thigh (bringing it back inward) after abducting it (raising it to the side while standing) may be caused by the tendon of the iliopsoas coming back over the hip joint capsule. It is not painful unless one has inflammation of the bursa *(bursa iliopectinea)* that lies in front of the hip joint and beneath the iliopsoas tendon. Also the tendon of the tensor fascia lata may snap forward over the greater trochanter of the femur as one makes sweeping semicircular movements with the lower limb or does squats with feet pointing out. This may indicate weakness of the thigh abductors. Such snapping is seldom painful but degeneration of the greater trochanter may result when it is experienced over a long period. To remedy this problem, strengthen the abductor muscles of the hip and stretch the tensor fascia lata—one of the abductors (Arnheim 1986).

Falls or blows to the outside of the hip can damage the superficial trochanteric bursa (a sack with fluid that lies between the greater trochanter and tensor fascia lata and prevents them from rubbing against each other). Major bleeding in the bursa may result in a clot that with time will change into adhesions or loose bodies. These adhesions and loose bodies can cause inflammation of the bursa and make creaking noises during hip movement. Inflammation of the bursa is very painful, even when one is not moving. See an orthopedic surgeon or a physician knowledgeable in applied kinesiology to make sure that all is okay.

Snapping sounds from the hip may be caused by the iliofemoral ligament moving over the head of the femur during either hip flexion or abduction.

Pain or Soreness and Stretching

I keep getting questions showing that the "no pain, no gain" fallacy still persists.

Question: I bought your book *Stretching Scientifically* and I am eager to try your method. I don't want to hurt my muscles and so decrease my flexibility. However, I am still not quite sure how to determine when I am not overstretching, especially during dynamic stretching and isometric stretching. What are some of the feelings or signs to tell when I have stretched enough for a particular set? If pain is one of them, does that mean I should stretch till it hurts every time?

Answer: You have stretched enough when you reach the maximal painless range of motion possible at the given stage of your training. In both dynamic and in static (isometric and relaxed) stretching you are overstretching if you feel pain. The in-depth answers to your question are on pages 31, 32, 51, 75 and 76.

Question: Should I feel a slight soreness the next day or two after isometric stretching (3 reps of 30 sec split holds, both front and side)? And since I do feel soreness after this activity what should I do to stretch isometrically without feeling pain in my muscles?

Answer: Slight soreness once in a while is to be expected in training but soreness occurring after every application of the same exercises, in your case isometric stretches, is a sign that you are not ready for these exercises. See pages 49–51 for how to prepare for isometric stretches.

Question: Can I do dynamic stretches when I am sore?

Answer: I think that you can do dynamic stretches such as relaxed leg raises and arm swings. I would do only as many repetitions and sets as I'd feel relaxing and not tiring.

Question: One year ago I had a ligament injury in my knee which took 6 months to heal. Also I met with an accident due to which I had to stop my training for 6 months. Now that I'm trying to come back, stretching is becoming very painful. Even with a minor stretch I experience ripping pain at the back of the knee. I was never good at stretching. I experience normal pain while stretching the left leg but I feel something tearing at the back of the right knee.

Is there a way I can improve my stretching even with a bad knee? Is it possible to do splits even with an a knee like mine?

Answer: A careful reading of *Stretching Scientifically* would tell you there is no such nonsense as "normal pain while stretching." If you stretch through pain you may achieve your splits but you will regret it later. Whether you can achieve splits with a bad knee depends on the exact nature of the injury, on effectiveness of rehabilitation, and on the rational method of flexibility training.

Question: Within the two months that I have been following your program my flexibility has improved a great deal. In the side split I am lower than I have ever been in all my [five] years of [karate] training. Upon receiving your videotape I stopped going to karate because I wanted to concentrate only on my splits. I did not want to go through the pain of stretching in class. In other words I did not want to mix the two different styles of stretching. Now that my flexibility has improved I started to attend karate workouts again and my joints are sore. When I kick I feel some pain, even when the kick is below the belt. Is this normal? I know for a fact that my joints are more tight than most people's. Is it possible to change this?

Answer: Regarding your question on the cause of joint pain or soreness after returning to karate training, I cannot give you a definite answer because I do not know enough about you and your training. Some of the possible causes may be:

a) poor kicking technique such as bad body alignment, not leaning back in roundhouse and side kicks (see the video *Power High Kicks with No Warm-Up!* for the proper technique and drills);

b) inadequate strength preparation (as shown and explained in the video *Secrets of Stretching*);

c) not enough (or wrong) dynamic stretching in the morning and later in the day (it has to be done twice a day, on workout days during your warm-up);

d) doing too much too soon; or

e) abnormal or injured joints (consult your doctor).

Question: Although the book and the video go into depth about stretching, I found that they did not fully explain the stretches to be performed by those who suffer from "weak knees." What strength exercises will strengthen the muscles that stabilize the knee?

Answer: If your knees hurt when you do a stretch, change it so your knee bears less or no weight. For example, in hamstring stretches or adductor stretches leading to a front or side split, place the lower end of your thigh on a chair or on any support. If bending your knees is not a problem you may do the exercise shown on the bottom of page 82.

The strength exercises that stabilize the knee are all those that affect muscles that originate above and attach below the knee joint. These exercises are squats, step-ups, deadlifts, and good mornings. If you cannot do these exercises because your knees were injured, then you can do isometric tensions with your knees held at angles at which you do not feel pain.

Question: My groin gets very sore when I do the side split exercises. Is there anything I can do about that?

Answer: Strengthen your inner thigh muscles.

Question: When I try to go down into the side splits I hurt very bad in my hips for up to 2 weeks. Is this normal?

Answer: It is to be expected if you are not ready for side splits and do not know how to position your pelvis. See pages 61 and 112 for information on the proper alignment of pelvis and thighs. If applying this information does not help, then see a doctor.

Question: After a hard squash game . . . my shoulder is sore and is becoming chronically sore. Also, my shoulder joints make all kinds of noises as I move my arms—creaks, snaps, pops, etc. It feels like ligaments and tendons are catching on things and then suddenly snapping free. This can't be normal, is it? So I am doing the stretching routine for the shoulders.

Answer: I do not believe that stretching your shoulders will help you. Soreness of your shoulder that becomes chronic can be caused by working out too often, by weakness of some muscles of the upper body that causes misalignment of the shoulder joint and thus forces some of its muscles to work inefficiently, and by overworking of the biceps brachii (which may cause swelling of its long head's tendon and grind against its groove in the arm bone).

Whenever ligaments or tendons "are catching on things," there is a possibility of inflammation and eventual damage to inflamed structures. An inflamed tendon of the long head of the biceps swells, rubs against the bony groove in which it moves, and pops out of it. As a result you get bone spurs in this groove. Also the ligament that holds the tendon in the groove gets overstretched so the tendon pops out of it easier and gets further aggravated. The bone spurs irritate the tendon and may eventually fry it.

Shoulder problems usually start with the impingement syndrome—when the biceps tendon or rotator cuff muscles are squeezed between the head of the arm bone and top parts of the shoulder blade (the coracoacromial arch). This impingement causes inflammation of the subacromial bursa and the muscles passing under the coracoacromial arch. Eventually you can get rotator cuff tears (partial or complete) and biceps tendon inflammation possibly ending with its complete tear or avulsion (detachment) from its origin. When your muscles and subacromial bursa are inflamed, the cartilage in your shoulder joint may also be inflamed and badly damaged (ripped and shredded to the point where it does not even resemble joint cartilage). You won't feel the damage to your joint cartilage until the joint mechanics change drastically because joint cartilage has no pain receptors.

Partial tears of muscles and bone spurs may require surgery to prevent more serious injuries to the joint and muscles. A surgical repair of a rotator cuff or biceps tear (often both are present) may put you out of your sport for at least six months if not forever. I suggest you read *Management of Common Musculoskeletal Disorders: Physical Therapy Principles and Methods* by Darlene Hertling and Randolph M. Kessler. This excellent book should help you evaluate qualifications of physical therapists or even design your own program of therapy.

Another cause of the swelling of the biceps tendon may be a digestive problem. In some digestive problems the lymphatic system is overwhelmed by toxins and cannot remove metabolic waste from tired muscles. Muscles then recover poorly and stay painful, weak, and sometimes tense. Digestive causes of your shoulder problems can be accurately diagnosed and removed by a doctor specializing in applied kinesiology. To find such a doctor in your area, visit http://www.icak.com.

Injuries and Stretching

Many people write to me with questions that can be summed up thus: "I have a boo-boo . . . I have overdone my exercises . . . I have torn this or broke that . . . what should I do now?" Being polite I answer to this effect: "I think you shouldn't be doing it, but now that you have done it, you should see a doctor." I have no clue why they think it makes sense to ask what to do of someone who has never seen them and who is not a physician but a physical education teacher. The best I know about treating injuries is this: *Look for the best specialist you can find and do not bother with people who do not come across as competent and fully committed to do the best that can be done. Then follow the doctor's orders without second-guessing. A good injury specialist can tell you in advance how your symptoms will change over time as you heal, when you will feel improvement, and how long it will take for full recovery.*

Question: One day while stretching in a taekwondo dojang [gym] in Korea, I was doing "butterflies" [see bottom picture on page 82]. When my instructor saw that my knees were not touching the floor, he came up behind me and forced them hard and quickly to the floor. The muscle was pulled in the left groin. Since then I have been very hesitant to stretch because of dull pain in that area. Maybe I'm doing something wrong?

Answer: Yes—you were doing something wrong. You were putting up with too much nonsense from a stupid "instructor." Now you should contact an applied kinesiologist or a very good orthopaedic surgeon and hope for the best. My experience with physicians specializing in applied kinesiology has been very good, and those that I have met are less conservative as far as exercise recommendations go and more knowledgeable, patient-oriented, and effective than all the "sports medicine specialists" that ever treated me.

To find Applied Kinesiology specialists practicing in U.S.A., Canada, Australia, New Zealand, and several countries of Europe and Asia, contact the International College of Applied Kinesiology

International College of Applied Kinesiology
6405 Metcalf Ave. Suite 503
Shawnee Mission, KS 66202
phone: 913-384-5336
fax: 913-384-5112
http://www.icak.com

If you have a choice, go to those doctors who are Diplomates of the International College of Applied Kinesiology and have initials DIBAK after their names. The safest course of action is to also see an orthopedic surgeon specializing in sports injuries.

Question: About 4 months ago I was stretching and injured the back of left leg. I was doing the splits with my left leg forward and tried to sink down farther than my body would allow. I felt a sudden "pop!" precisely where my leg meets my butt. I felt a dull pain but thought I would be okay. I couldn't run or walk fast for a long time. Now 4 months later I can run but the injury still persists. Sometimes I have a dull pain in the area or feel some discomfort. What might this injury be and do you have any advice?

Answer: Feeling a pop indicates that you had a third or fourth degree strain (muscle tear). This is serious damage—many muscle fibers are completely torn, fascia is damaged (in the fourth degree strain the fascia, and so the whole muscle, is torn apart). The gap in the muscle is filled with blood. The blood clots and is then replaced with a stiff scar. The bigger the clot the greater the scar, the loss of muscle's function, and the likelihood of repeat injury. Internal clots can also calcify—turn into sharp bonelike bodies—and keep cutting the surrounding muscle tissue. To minimize the damage, muscle strains must be taken care of immediately. If not, the loss of muscle strength and elasticity may be such that full function will never be regained and further injuries will occur because of it.

You say that after four months the injury still persists, so I assume that it was not treated by a medical professional. (If it had been, you would be fully recovered by now.) After four months of neglect there is little chance of regaining most of the pre-injury function. If your muscle was torn completely, by now nothing can be done—stitching and reattaching is done within two weeks of the strain. If it was not torn completely, then maybe it needs removal of the excessive scar tissue or of calcification. To see what you can do to regain what function you can, see an orthopedic surgeon and a physician specializing in applied kinesiology. I wrote extensively on muscle strains in the Winter 2002 issue of *Stadion News*, which you can download from http://www.stadion.com/freebies.html. In any case, do not dream that stretching is the solution to your problem.

Question: You say not to exercise until an injury or problem is totally solved. Does that mean avoiding stretching routines until a joint is healed?

Answer: Unless told by a doctor otherwise, I would avoid all exercise with strong tension of muscles around that joint as well as any movements at the maximum range of motion. This may still leave slow dynamic stretches, static active stretches, and gentle relaxed static passive stretches available to you.

Question: I was doing very well for about a month following your method. Then I tried adding the front split isometrics after completing my four sets of 30-second side splits and I strained my gracilis muscle. It seemed that I just overworked it. Any suggestions?

Answer: Your gracilis could have been exhausted by the four sets of isometric stretches for the side split, and so the following isometric stretch for the front split was more than it could take. It is worth knowing that the gracilis is weakened by adrenal stress that can arise from work or family stress or from training loads exceeding one's ability to adapt.

To speed up recovery and to have a chance of regaining full strength and function in cases of muscle strains or ligament sprains, I recommend seeing immediately a doctor who knows applied kinesiology. A good applied kinesiologist will be able to help you recover from this injury and possibly teach you how to avoid it in the future.

Question: I just recently pulled a hamstring in my right leg doing the front split. I rest it for a while till the pain is gone, but it is the same thing all over again when I resume isometric stretches.

Answer: Absence of pain does not mean that recovery is complete. When the pain is gone the rehabilitation begins—and that is a long way from being ready for the pre-injury level of activity. Another possible cause for the recurrence of your muscle strain is that resting your injured hamstring does not remove the cause of the injury. Here is my advice:

a) See an applied kinesiologist or an orthopedic surgeon concerning your hamstring (or whatever injury) and do what your doctor advises you to do.

b) When permitted by your doctor, start doing the following exercises in this order: walking, climbing stairs, running uphill, squats, hamstring curls, stiff-legged deadlifts (or other exercises appropriate for whatever muscles you have to rehabilitate). Progress from one exercise to another only when feeling no discomfort performing the previous one.

c) Only after complete recovery (when hamstrings or other injured muscles of both legs are equally strong, equally flexible, and have equal endurance) can you try isometric stretches involving those muscles.

Question: After reading about your stretching technique in a magazine I decided to get your book *Stretching Scientifically* and see if it would work for me. I started in and got to isometric splits. Things were going okay for a while and suddenly I felt my groin muscle give way and a lot of pain. I guessed that I tore a muscle and it took about two weeks before I stopped feeling pain in my groin. I put the book back on the shelf (after that experience who wouldn't) and decided to pick it back up tonight. Well, once again, I got to isometric splits. I started really high (almost in a wide leg stance with my legs straight) and tensed my inner thighs. Without warning I felt a pop and again the pain returned. Now my groin hurts standing normally and when pulling thighs to the inside. I'm 18 and I love weightlifting. What have I been doing wrong? Every time I've tried isometric stretches I've torn something and it's taken me out of commission. There must be some way to correct what I'm doing wrong and achieve full (or even close to full) splits.

Answer: What have you been doing wrong? I suspect that you have not gone through the exercise program of preparing for isometric stretches that is described at the beginning of chapter 5, "Isometric Stretches," on pages 49 and 50. The same program of exercises will help with the final stages of rehabilitating your muscle tears.

You write that you love weightlifting. Do you do most of your lifts explosively or with near maximal weights? If so, you may be capable of tensing your muscles very strongly and very quickly. If you do that with muscles of the inner thigh, which most people do not exercise for strength and muscular endurance in adduction movements, you can tense them harder than their structure can withstand and rip them. (If you tense a muscle or pull on it very quickly, its tendon—if healthy—stiffens and so the energy is absorbed mostly by the muscle's belly, which stretches or tears—depending on the amount of the energy.)

Other causes: Muscles that are tired or inflamed are easier to tear than well-rested and healthy muscles. If you take steroids, or supplements that increase the force of your muscles' contractions, the structural strength of the muscles may lag behind their contractile strength and muscle belly or even tendon tears are likely.

It is bad to tear a muscle. It is much worse to tear it again. You can find out the nature of your injury and how to fully rehabilitate it by studying books on injuries that are listed at The Athlete's Bookshelf (http://www.stadion.com/bookshelf.html). I especially recommend *Management of Common Musculoskeletal Disorders: Physical Therapy Principles and Methods* because this book explains how to rehabilitate after an injury as well as what the lifetime consequences are of not letting an injured muscle heal, not rehabilitating it fully, and reinjuring it. Another title I recommend is *Complementary Sports Medicine.*

Question: I got your book *Stretching Scientifically* a while back and have seen great progress. However, I've developed an injury to my pectineus muscle on my inner left thigh. I injured it some time back; exactly how I injured it or what I did to injure it, I truly don't remember. It's been nagging me for a while, and when I try to do the side split it positively kills me with pain. I was down to about 1–2 inches off the floor, before the pain from this injury came back and prevented any serious further attempts. I paid my first visit to an applied kinesiologist today. The doctor pointed to a strained (or possibly slightly torn) left pectineus. He suggested replacing my running program with lots of swimming, frequent icing, no weight exercises at all, and laying off the stretching. I guess I have two questions:

1. In your experience, does this sound reasonable, or perhaps do you know of any other exercises I can try?

2. I was so close to the side split. I can wait a while longer to allow an injury to heal, but in a general sense I guess I'm asking . . . is there hope? Will I ever be able to do it?

Answer: Yes, it sounds very reasonable. I do not second-guess a physician specializing in Applied Kinesiology who has examined you. If you want to keep stretching before your pectineus heals you will cripple yourself for good.

Do not be so eager to preserve your "pride and joy"—your near-side split stretch—at the risk of a permanent injury. First heal completely, then rehabilitate carefully, and then start working out and stretching—after all with the right stretching method, the silly side split takes only from a few weeks to a few months.

Question: I am fifty-one years old, in good shape. For several years I have noticed that my right leg is much tighter than the left and recently I have noticed definite pain in the middle of the right buttock that also radiates down the leg. A week ago I was doing a static hamstring stretch sitting on the floor when I felt a stab of pain across my lower back. I have had pretty bad spasms ever since and I have trouble straightening up after sitting. Do you have any suggestions as to how can I overcome this and get back to training?

Answer: It looks like you have a lower back problem that was developing for several years—even before you first noticed that your right leg is tighter than the left. To find out when and if you can exercise again see an applied kinesiologist. The referral number of the International College of Kinesiology is on page 165.

Question: I have recently recovered from a low-back strain and have been told to do sit-ups, back extensions, and leg extensions to keep the muscles in this area strong. I would like to know if doing these exercises after my morning stretch would defeat the purpose of the dynamic and relaxed stretches?

Answer: No, these exercises would not ruin the effect of the stretches. To maximize the effect of both exercises and the stretches, you may start your morning with dynamic stretches, then do the exercises for your back, and then do relaxed stretches.

Question: On page 63 you state that people who experience knee problems should do strength exercises. What are these strength exercises?

Answer: Climbing stairs, squats, and deadlifts.

Question: What sort of injury could result from doing the side split, toes up position? I believe that my thigh was not rotated enough while I was very close to the ground; when I rotated my toes more to the ceiling I felt a popping in my left hip. Subsequent to this I have experienced extremely sharp pain (which I assume is the result of nerve damage of some sort) ever since. The pain in sitting runs from my sit bones [ischium] through my hamstring and into the calf and ankle areas. The injury was almost a year ago, and the pain of sitting is the worst but it has subsided—at first I could only sit for 10 minutes before having to get up, now it is an hour. I have dutifully done physiotherapy exercises and submitted myself to chiropractic treatment, and I have had my pelvis x-rayed (no problem there). Specialists can find nothing wrong except to say that it could be pressure on the sciatic nerve. I took plenty of time off immediately after the injury and slowly introduced my martial arts and stretching routine again. All of this, and it is still not healed. Do you have any suggestions?

Answer: To do a side split with toes up one has to start spreading the legs while sitting and not slide into this split. You would not get into this trouble if you had used the stretches shown in the *Stretching Scientifically*.

It seem like the specialists that you have seen are right and the sciatic nerve is pressed or irritated by something. To find out what causes the irritation and what to do about it you need to see someone who knows how to treat musculoskeletal injuries.

Question: You recommend avoiding relaxed lower back stretches in a standing position so as not to stretch ligaments. Unfortunately, when I first started training in martial arts the standing toe touch was one of the most common stretches and I didn't know any better at the time as I was unaware of your methods.

Is there any way of knowing whether you have stretched the ligaments of the spine and are there any corrective exercises that can reshorten them? Furthermore, can hanging from a bar, as in hanging leg raises, also stretch lower back ligaments?

Answer: To find out whether you have stretched the ligaments of the spine, see an orthopedic surgeon. Overstretched ligaments may be associated with back pain because of hypermobility of back joints or because of entrapment of the tissues that normally would be kept out of the joint by the ligaments (Hertling and Kessler 1996).

I do not know if it is possible to fully reshorten the overstretched ligaments. With age, ligaments of the spine become shorter, but so do the vertebral disks, and the end result may be ligamentous laxity and back pain from the causes given above. Rehabilitation of overstretched ligaments consists of refraining from stretching them and doing strength exercises for the muscles supporting the spine. In time, the ligaments may regain some of their integrity (Hertling and Kessler 1996).

Unless you already have weakened ligaments and muscles of the back, hanging from a bar should not overstretch them. For healthy people, hanging from a bar does not put such stress on the ligaments as bending forward with a hunched back. It is like pulling on a stick versus bending it.

No Success

Many problems described here arise from not paying attention to what is written in this book and from neglecting strength training/preparation prior to starting intensive stretching program.

Question: I tried to determine my flexibility potential for a side split. I can't tilt the pelvis forward *and* rotate my thigh outward. If I can't do that, then do I have a hip structure problem or is it just that my hip ligaments are very tight? What should I do to overcome this problem?

Answer: I think that you have misunderstood the side split test. It seems that you tried to simultaneously tilt your pelvis forward and rotate your thigh outward. That must be really difficult. I tried it and I could not do it either.

The test does not require tilting your pelvis forward—only rotating your thigh and raising it to the hip level. Read pages 109–111 carefully and do the test *as shown*.

Question: I have been using isometric stretches for the front and side splits for three months and had made some progress, although not as much as I would have liked. However, recently I seem to have "hit the wall" so to speak and can progress no further. I am still ten inches from a front split and 14 inches from a side split. I have done the "split test" and have the right range of motion. Are weak adductors holding me back, and would adductor flies be the best method of targeting these areas? My overall leg strength is very good otherwise.

Answer: If indeed you pass both split tests (tests of hip joints mobility and thigh muscles' length) then "hitting the wall" may be caused by weakness of the muscles stretched in the splits (thigh adductors, psoas, hamstrings), so strengthening them may help. In your strength workouts do squats, front and side lunges, deadlifts, and good mornings. Make sure you do your strength exercises in the full range of motion. "Hitting the wall" may also be caused by doing the isometric stretches all the time the same old way—with the same amount of tension, in the same body alignment, on the same surface. Try tensing harder, leaning your trunk and bending knees more or less, and stretching on more or less slippery surface, perhaps even sliding up and down in stretched out stances.

Question: I have your book *Stretching Scientifically* and the video. I believe that my problem is my hip. As a child I dislocated my hip and have been more flexible in one leg than the other. When I do the stretching exercises, I feel pain in my hips before I even begin to feel any type of stretch in my leg muscles. When I first start to do a side split I can only move my feet apart 2–3 feet until I get warmed up, and the tightness is from my hips. When I sit to do butterflies my legs do not even come close to touching the floor. Is there anything that you can tell me to help?

Answer: Your problem is addressed on pages 61 and 62 in chapter 5, "Isometric Stretching," and on pages 111 and 112 in chapter 8, "All the Whys of Stretching." If you can align the hips and thighs as shown on the Test of Flexibility Potential then all you need to do is to strengthen and stretch the muscles controlling your hip joints by practicing your stretches in positions shown on those pages. If even with a good warm-up you cannot perform the Test of Flexibility Potential then perhaps the structure of your hip joints (the length and angulation of the neck of your thigh) does not allow sufficient mobility for a side split. In that case you better stop trying before you injure your hips.

The fact that the tightness of your hips is relieved by warming up may mean that the cause of tightness is a soft tissue resistance rather than the bone structure. To find out for sure see either a good orthopedic surgeon or a physician specializing in Applied Kinesiology.

Question: I am twenty years old and am extremely inflexible, particularly in the shoulders and hips. I have been interested in and worked at martial arts off and on for the past three years, but as much I want to be good at it, I am always disheartened by my inflexibility. I am almost positive that I do not have, and never have had, normal joint rotation, and I cannot do the side-split test in *Stretching Scientifically* while keeping my hips and raised leg in a straight line. The book assumes that most people would pass this test and says nothing about what do to if someone does not have "normal" range of motion in their hip joints. I realize that since the book does not mention it, I probably will never be able to have full, proper joint rotation, but I just want to improve it as much as possible, not necessarily for martial arts, but most importantly for my health.

Answer: If you do the side-split test properly and cannot pass it, then you may not have normal mobility of your hip joints. If the mobility of your hip joints is limited by their bone structure, then you will not be able to do the full side split. Still, if you keep working on your flexibility (but without forcing your joints), you may achieve a greater range and ease of motion than if you don't.

Question: Is it possible to increase the outside rotation of the thigh with strength and/or stretching exercises?

Answer: That depends what limits the outside rotation of the thigh. It may be limited by the bone structure of your hip joint (nothing can be done about that), or tightness of soft tissues (ligaments and muscles—this can be worked on). If ligaments at the front of the hip joint restrict your range of outside rotation and abduction, then flexing the hip joint (leaning your trunk forward) should let you spread your legs wider because it relaxes those ligaments. If the muscles that resist outward rotation are too short, then exercises may elongate them. Try sumo squats or ballet squats (with feet pointing out, but without twisting the knees!) and stretches in positions of maximal outward rotation of the thigh or combined maximal outward rotation and abduction of the thigh.

A sample initial position for a stretch for outside (external) rotation of the thigh: lie face down, bend one knee 90 degrees so the shin is vertical, let that shin fall inward and down so it is as close as possible to the other, straight leg.

A sample initial position for a stretch for combined outward rotation and abduction of the thigh: sit in half lotus (half Indian squat), grab the ankle of the bent leg so you can pull it up, put the other hand on the knee of the bent leg so you can push it down.

Another option is to patiently work on the horse-riding stance— starting high and with feet only shoulder -width apart and gradually progressing lower and then wider. Just make sure that your stance is perfect, with your thighs parallel to the floor at any width, toes pointing forward, and chest up. The wider and lower your stance, the more forward you will have to tilt your pelvis. At all stages (heights, widths) you must be able to do deep and calm abdominal breathing. If you rush and progress to wider and deeper stances before becoming comfortable at the current stage you may hurt your knees, subluxate or fix your sacrum, and get lower back and neck pains.

Question: I am finding it quite difficult to assume the half lotus position (used for meditation in Shorinji Kempo [a martial art]) although I am very close to being able to do full side and front splits.

I wonder if you could recommend any stretches or strength exercises to help me get into the lotus position?

Answer: To increase the range of abduction and external rotation in the hip, try using the stretch at the bottom of page 82. It can be made more effective by putting sandbags on your thighs close to your bent knees. You can also stretch one thigh at a time, sitting with one leg straight in front of you and the other bent with its ankle resting on the thigh of the straight leg. In such a half-butterfly stretch press your bent knee down with your arm or use a sandbag to increase range of motion and provide resistance as in isometric stretches. I think it is not a good idea to increase your range of motion by stretching the ligaments of your ankles and knees as this will predispose you to injuries. It is better not to do the lotus position right than to have lax ligaments. Also, I have noticed that the people who can do lotus position do not have much muscle mass on their thighs. Slim thighs may make it easier to cross the legs and put the tops of feet or ankles on the thighs than massive thighs.

Question: I have tried your stretching methods and I find that the tension in my adductors is great and I cannot really get any closer to the floor in the side splits position. (Sliding down from the horse-riding stance I am at least 16 inches [40 centimeters] from the floor.)

Having done sprints for 17-odd years and 10 years of weights (including power lifting and Olympic lifting movements) I know I have the strength but find I am currently stuck. I cannot do the side-split test and have my foot pointing upwards; as I move to try and have my hips in line, my foot wants to point to the side. I can get quite low doing a front split but have a little trouble getting the hips to straighten.

I'm not quite sure if I have reached as far as I can go. Is it just my body?

Answer: What is the maximal range of outside rotation of your thigh (see bottom photo on page 110 in *Stretching Scientifically*)? If it is less than 50 degrees in the hip joint (or less than 70 degrees of foot turnout), then perhaps that is what keeps you from sliding lower into the side split. The fact that your foot turns inward during the side-split test seems to indicate that you do not have enough range of motion in the outside rotation. This may be caused by the bone structure of your hip joint, or tightness of your soft tissues—ligaments and muscles. For solutions see my answer to the preceding question.

Your strength from sprinting and lifting weights may be specific for the sprinting and lifting movements you have done but not for standing in the very wide stances when thigh adductors have to tense in a near maximal stretch. Doing sumo squats, ballet squats, deep front and side lunges, and the horse-riding stance should improve your adductors' ability to support your weight in wide straddle stances.

By having "a little trouble getting the hips to straighten" in the front split, I assume you mean keeping the pelvis from tilting forward (keeping hips from flexing). If so, then you try to do the near impossible. In the front split the pelvis should be tilted forward, toward the front leg.

Question: I am a 36-year-old martial artist who has been practicing about eight years. I have been an athlete all my life, and have used many strength and stretching techniques. Your methods have been the most effective for me. After using your methods I find my kicks are stronger than before and I can "recall" my maximum stretch with very little warm-up. The problem I seem to have now is that I have reached a "sticking point" in my side splits and can't get further down than what you show in the top photos on page 63. I maintain my body in the upright position when doing side splits and don't use my hands for balance. I usually do three to five sets holding each tension for 20–30 seconds and concentrate on strength gains as you suggest. I have reread your book several times and it appears to me that I'm using your methods correctly. Why, then, can't I progress beyond the sticking point?

Answer: The cause of a sticking point may be any one of the following:

a) lack of strength of all muscles of the thigh (try low squats, one-legged squats, deadlifts, adductor flys, adductor pulldowns);

b) not tilting pelvis forward while spreading legs into a split, as shown on pages 61, 63, and 112. (Your pelvis moves on the axis joining both hip joints. A forward tilt makes the inlet of the pelvis face front more than in a natural position, a backward tilt makes it face more upward.);

c) not getting enough rest between workouts (see the *Science of Sports Training* for methods of evaluating sufficiency of recovery or readiness for working out); or

d) doing isometric exercises too often (2–4 times per week is enough).

Question: I am stuck at my current flexibility range. I'm a bit sore after my isometric stretches, I don't have any sharp pains, my muscles just feel stiff. I feel this soreness in the area above my thighs [in front of my pelvis]; my inner thighs don't bother me. In adductor flyes I currently use a weight boot with about 12 lb. on each foot. I use 27 lb. for the adductor pulldown load.

Answer: Your problem may have to do with weakness of your psoas muscles—the soreness in front of your pelvis indicates it. It may be caused by overworking them, by not having sufficiently strengthened them with leg raises before starting adductor exercises (see the video *Secrets of Stretching*), or by a wrong diet. This may be checked by very specific tests of Applied Kinesiology.

Question: I am almost twenty years old, in good shape, and exercise regularly, and eat very well. I can reach a front split almost perfectly with no warm-up, but my range of motion in a side split is only a little over ninety degrees. After jogging and then stretching isometrically for thirty minutes, including holding my side split with no hands for two minutes, my range of motion increases significantly (about nine inches off the floor), however, the next day my flexibility is as if I had never stretched at all.

Answer: The fact that you can get so close to the side split (only nine inches above the floor), even though it takes a long session of stretching, means that the most likely limitation of your ROM prior to this session and on the day after is the weakness of your muscles and not the structure of your hip joints. I recommend that you follow the whole program of strength exercises for hips and thighs that especially emphasizes the muscles that limit sideways motion in the hip joint, shown on the video *Secrets of Stretching.*

If you stretch isometrically for 30 minutes then no wonder you cannot make progress. Doing this much strenuous effort is counterproductive. Look at the video *Secrets of Stretching* and see how and for how long the stretches are done.

Also, consider if the jogging that you do prior to stretching is too intensive or too long. As I mention in *Stretching Scientifically,* fatiguing endurance work should not be done before strength efforts. Aerobic endurance work should not be done before strength efforts for reasons explained in the *Science of Sports Training,* but light aerobic efforts can be engaged in after any strenuous efforts (speed, strength, anaerobic endurance) as a means of speeding up recovery. This is why most of the sample workouts shown in *Stretching Scientifically* end with marching or jumping rope.

Do you start your isometric stretch for a side split from the position shown on page 61 or on page 63 and in the video *Secrets of Stretching*? If not, then you may be overstraining your thigh adductors so they cannot recover fully between workouts and so you are stuck at the same range of motion.

Impatience

So many ask "Are we there yet? How much longer?" as if they had no experience with any physical training and no sense of its effects on their bodies.

Question: I am within one foot of doing a complete side split. How do you feel when you can do it? I mean do you one day start your isometrics and go down all the way to a full side split for the first time? Is there anything else I can do to get over the hump and be able to do the side split?

Answer: You will notice that you slide lower and can stand lower or in a wider straddle without much change in the effort and without discomfort. To "get over the hump" keep training and let small changes accumulate until you find to be easy what was once difficult.

Question: What determines the speed of progress in stretching?

Answer: The speed of progress in stretching depends on your initial strength level and initial flexibility level, and on how rational your total training program is. Normally it takes well under a year to develop the ability to perform splits. I would like to take this opportunity to give you one essential training tip: Consider isometric stretches to be *strength* exercises and apply them as such. Use sufficient rest between workouts. Do not do more exercises than you need, i.e., do not do more than two isometric stretches per workout (you may do a few repetitions of a stretch but do not do many various stretches). Do not overwork any group of muscles.

Question: When can I expect to do a side split via isometric stretches without a warm-up? I have been able to do a side split at the end of my isometric workout for about two months now, but it takes about 3 sets of stretches to get that far down and I still start from nearly the same height above the floor.

Answer: The reasons for you having to warm up before you can do a full side split may be that:

1. Your exercises, although effective enough to let you do the side split, did not have enough time to change the muscles of your legs as much as it takes to do splits without any warm-up; or

2. Your body has not "learned" yet that sliding into a split is safe. (This possibility cannot be considered separately from the first one.)

In my experience an instant split (with isometric stretch or without it) can take from a couple of months to a few months after being capable of doing a full split.

I would advise doing heavy squats, lunges, and deadlifts (normal and sumo) until you can lift weights heavier than your body weight in the squat and about twice the body weight in deadlifts, and using isometric tensions to raise up from the straddle stance (extremely low horse-riding stance), and ultimately from the side split.

Question: What are the possible causes of inconsistency in flexibility? My own flexibility is often very inconsistent. From week to week, sometimes even day to day, it varies anywhere from near split to that of a rank beginner. I seem to have the worst flexibility and most soreness a day or two after a particularly good kick workout in which my legs were very limber and relatively free of pain.

Answer: You say "relatively free of pain." Does this mean that most of the time your legs hurt? If so, no wonder your flexibility suffers—tired or hurt muscles are less flexible than rested and healthy ones. From what you say it seems that the inconsistency in the level of flexibility you display is caused by irrational training. You do not have enough strength and muscular endurance for your kicking workouts and so after such a workout you are sore and inflexible.

Question: I'd like to ask you why after achieving a great stretch my muscles seem to tighten again. For example, I get myself into a full lotus, and then for a whole week after I can't get even close to it.

Answer: I think that there are two possible reasons for your problem:

1. You may be overstretching your muscles.

2. You may be overworking them with other exercises.

Question: You indicate that soreness after isometric exercises is the result of overdoing the exercises. After an isometric workout, I can really "feel" the muscles of my hamstrings and inner thighs when I flex them, but there is no pain. Does this mean I am over-training?

Answer: It depends how long after the workout you feel the soreness. Use the same judgment as you would in the case of lifting weights.

Question: In the event that I train my hip flexors or glutei very hard, and they feel tired or sore, should I skip dynamic stretches since I would use those muscles to raise my legs?

Answer: Usually not, if you do dynamic stretches correctly, but ultimately it depends on how sore you get. You should not be in such a poor shape as to have difficulties with a few leg raises next day after a hard workout.

Question: When one has a couple of days off—due to muscle soreness or just rest days—does it cause flexibility to decrease and set one back in training schedule?

Answer: Flexibility usually does not decrease much, and may even increase because of the rest the muscles got. If you do isometric stretches or any strength exercises even when you are sore because you are so anxious not to lose your flexibility temporarily, you may injure yourself and lose it permanently. You can do relaxed stretches, however, even if your muscles are sore as long as doing these stretches does not cause pain.

Question: I've been using your techniques for a month now, with good improvement when I slide down into a side split. However, when I sit down and try to spread my legs into a straddle there doesn't seem to be any improvement there. Why is this?

Answer: The reasons why you can stretch your legs further while standing in a straddle stance than while sitting are these:

1. To slide down from a straddle stance you use alternating tensions and relaxations to suppress your stretch reflex and so to slide your legs further apart. When you are sitting you do not tense your

inner thighs and even if you wanted to there is nothing to give you an adequate resistance.

2. When you stand, the muscles of your thighs are tensed and so the stretch reflex may be depressed. (During an isometric tension the stretch reflex is depressed.) When you are sitting your thighs are relaxed and so the stretch reflex is not depressed.

3. You have used isometric stretches for only a month and that is not enough time to show much improvement in your range of motion in a static active stretch. (Spreading legs while sitting, with no pressure against the inside of the legs, amounts to a static active stretch.)

Question: I have been trying for a couple of months to do the side split. My problem is that I still seem to be about the same distance off the floor now as I was then.

My training routine consists of going to the gym 3–4 times a week and lifting weights for all parts of the body. I do squats, leg curls, lunges, and hack squats for my legs. Then when I go home and just before I go to bed at night I do the 100 reps [of adductor flys] for the inside of my leg and then I do the isometric exercises for the side split.

Answer: You may be doing too much. If you do 100 adductor flyes and isometric stretches every evening, or even just on the evenings after lifting weights in the gym, then no wonder you have tight hips and other problems. At least four times per week you are doing two strength workouts for the same muscle groups on the same day—if you lift serious weights it is only a matter of a short time before you get injured.

You may need to decrease or increase the resistance, or change the frequency of your workouts—depending on your reaction. For methods of matching your training to your recovery see *Science of Sports Training.*

Stretching Machines
and Other Strange Practices

Question: I have heard it said by many martial artists that staying in a full side split for hours at a time increases flexibility. Is this true or just a myth?

Answer: Judge it yourself. What do they have to show for it?

Question: Can a stretching machine be used to aid stretching?

Answer: There is no need for using stretching machines. In relaxed stretches for the hips and thighs, you can as easily relax into a stretch on your own on a smooth floor. If you try doing isometric stretches for hips and thighs in a stretching machine, the machine will make it more difficult for you to tense your muscles because it prevents the weight of your body from pressing on your thighs and thus forcing them to tense more. The harder you tense in isometric stretches, the greater is the following relaxation and the resulting stretch.

In my 25 years of living in Poland I have not seen even one stretching machine and I worked out in the best equipped training halls in Warsaw (at AWF—the University School of Physical Education), and in several other cities. I didn't see a stretching machine anywhere because athletes do not need stretching machines. (Actually, I have never heard or seen any mention of stretching machines in any country of the Soviet Bloc. I think there was not a single stretching machine in the whole Soviet Bloc—who would need it?)

For able-bodied persons the stretching machines are a waste of money as simple stretches on the floor do just as well or better.

If you want to stretch the muscles of your shoulders and arms, then a rope with knots held behind your back and worked with your hands like a rosary or prayer beads is all you need.

Stretching machines "may be particularly helpful for special populations, such as the elderly and those with physical problems that prevent them from executing certain stretches by themselves" ("Stretching Machines" 1999). Unless you have been severely injured or have a crippling disease, you do not need a machine to increase your flexibility. Manufacturers of stretching machines know it too. The editors of *Georgia Tech Sports Medicine & Performance Newsletter* report a study of stretching machines conducted at the University of Oregon and funded by a company that manufactures stretching machines. The study showed flexibility gains among people who stretched on the machines *but their gains were not compared to the people who stretched without machines* ("Stretching Machines" 1999).

Other

Question: What is the difference between your book and your video on stretching? Do I need the video? Should I buy your video to get my full flexibility?

Answer: Stretching methods shown in the book and on the video are the same. The book shows stretches for the whole body. It only mentions but does not show exercises other than stretches that develop strength and endurance while promoting flexibility. The book tells you all that you must know about flexibility but you have to devise your own exercise program on the basis of the provided (and abundant) information.

The video shows stretches as well as recommended endurance and strength exercises for your legs and trunk. The video is of the "do-along" type. If you do not know much about strength training, if your flexibility suffers because of lack of strength, if doing stretches makes your back tired, if you are often sore after a workout—then the video may help you.

Question: Why don't you make a video for athletes who have a particular level of flexibility, for example, those who cannot reach their toes?

Answer: This method works regardless of anybody's level of flexibility. Exercises are demonstrated at a fairly high range of motion, but one can do them at any range, no matter how low, and increase it gradually.

Resources for Further Study

Science of Sports Training: How to Plan and Control Training for Peak Performance by Thomas Kurz (Island Pond, VT: Stadion Publishing Company), 2001.

This comprehensive text delves deeply into topics such as speeding up recovery, using time- and energy-efficient training methods, avoiding overtraining and injuries, applying proven methods of training to specific sports, and maintaining a high level of condition and skills for years. You will learn ways to plan and control training for each workout, over a span of years.

Secrets of Stretching: Exercises for the Lower Body (VHS videotape, 98 min.), featuring Tom Kurz (Island Pond, VT: Stadion Publishing Company), 1990.

This video features an introduction to general conditioning and follows that with four exercise routines—one for beginners, one for intermediate, and two for advanced athletes. You will learn plenty of how-tos. The focus is on combining flexibility training with strength training.

Power High Kicks with No Warm-Up! (VHS videotape, 80 min.), featuring Mac Mierzejewski (Island Pond, VT: Stadion Publishing Company), 1996.

This video teaches everything there is to know about kicks: body alignments that allow kicking high and with power without any warm-up, footwork, drills, and developing power. Simple exercises make sure that your hips and knees don't hurt when you throw high side and roundhouse kicks. You will learn the "little" details of kicking techniques that let you kick high and with power without a warm-up while at the same time reducing your chance of injury!

Explosive Power and Jumping Ability for All Sports: Atlas of Exercises by Tadeusz Starzynski and Henryk Sozanski (Island Pond, VT: Stadion Publishing Company), 1999.

How well you jump and how powerfully you punch, pull, or throw depends on your explosive power, on your special endurance for explosive movements, and on your speed, coordination, and flexibility. *Explosive Power and Jumping Ability for All Sports* tells you how to develop each of these abilities.

Children and Sports Training: How Your Future Champions Should Exercise to Be Healthy, Fit, and Happy by Józef Drabik (Island Pond, VT: Stadion Publishing Company), 1996.

Here is what Lyle J. Micheli, M.D., Director of Sports Medicine at Children's Hospital, Boston; President of the American College of Sports Medicine; and Fellow of the American Academy of Pediatrics said about this book:

"This book represents the cumulative knowledge and experience of the author and many of his [East European] colleagues related to the progressive preparation and training for children in organized sports."

Appendix A: Hip Joint and Shoulder Joint in Abduction

The following photographs taken by Prof. Ciszek and Dr. Smigielski (1997) show configuration of the bones and ligaments of the hip joint and the shoulder joint in pure abduction and in abduction with external rotation.

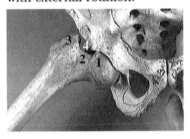

Fig. 1. Bones of the hip joint in maximal abduction—front view
1. femoral head
2. femoral neck
3. greater trochanter
4. roof of joint socket

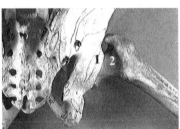

Fig. 2. Bones of the hip joint in maximal abduction—back view
1. roof of joint socket
2. femoral neck

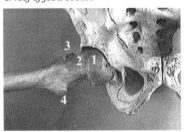

Fig. 3. Bones of the hip joint in abduction with external rotation—front view
1. femoral head
2. femoral neck

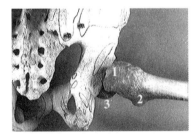

Fig. 4. Bones of the hip joint in abduction with external rotation—back view
1. greater trochanter
2. lesser trochanter
3. femoral head

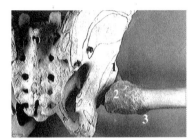

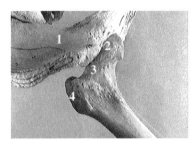

Fig. 5. Bones of the hip joint in abduction
with more external rotation—back view
1. roof of joint socket
2. greater trochanter
3. lesser trochanter

Fig. 6. Bones of the hip joint in abduction
with external rotation—top view
1. iliac fossa
2. femoral head
3. femoral neck
4. greater trochanter

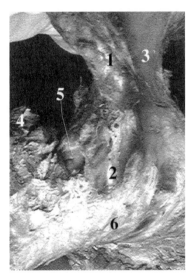

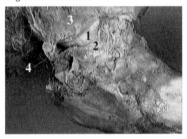

Fig. 8. Hip joint in maximal abduction—
back view
1. femoral head
2. capsule
3. roof of joint socket
4. free space in the joint cavity

Fig. 7. Bones, cartilage, and ligaments of
the hip joint in maximal abduction—front
view
1. iliac crest
2. insertion of rectus femoris
3. iliac fossa
4. greater trochanter
5. labrum acetabulare
6. pubofemoral ligament
7. femoral neck

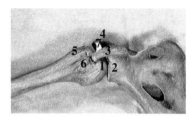 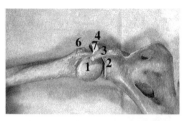

Fig. 9. Bones of the shoulder joint in glenohumeral abduction—front view
1. head of humerus
2. rim of the glenoid cavity
3. coracoid process
4. acromion process
5. greater tubercle
6. lesser tubercle
7. coraco-acromial ligament

Fig. 10. Bones of the shoulder joint in abduction with external rotation—front view
1. head of humerus
2. rim of the glenoid cavity
3. coracoid process
4. acromion
5. greater tubercle
6. lesser tubercle
7. coraco-acromial ligament

Appendix B: Normal Range of Motion

(Kapandji 1974, 1982, 1987; Potter 1986)

Neck
Extension 55° . . . . Try to point up with chin.
Flexion 40° . . . . Touch sternum with chin.
Lateral bending 35° . . . . Bring ear close to shoulder.
Rotation 70° left and right . . . . Turn head far to the left, then right.
Lumbar Spine
Extension 30° . . . . Bend backward.
Flexion 60° . . . . Bend forward at the waist.
Lateral bending 20° . . . . Bend to the side.
Shoulder
Abduction 180° . . . . Bring arm sideways up.
Adduction 30°–45° . . . . Bring arm toward the midline of the body.
Horizontal extension 30°–40° . . . . Swing arm horizontally backward.
Horizontal flexion 130° . . . . Swing arm horizontally forward.
Vertical extension 45°–50° . . . . Raise arm straight backward.
Vertical flexion 180° . . . . Raise arm straight forward.
External rotation 80° . . . . Bend arm and move forearm away from abdomen.
Internal rotation 110° . . Bend arm and bring forearm behind and away from back.
Elbow
Extension 180° . . . . Straighten out lower arm.
Flexion 150° . . . . Bring lower arm to the biceps.
Pronation 80°–85° . . . . Turn lower arm so palm faces down.
Supination 90° . . . . Turn lower arm so palm of the hand faces up.
Wrist
Extension 70° . . . . . . Bend wrist so back of hand nears outer surface of lower arm.
Flexion 80°–90° . . . . Bend wrist so palm nears inner surface of lower arm.
Radial deviation 15° . . . . Bend wrist so thumb nears radius.
Ulnar deviation 30°–50° . . . . Bend wrist so small finger nears ulna.
Hip
Extension 30° . . . . Move thigh backward without moving pelvis.
Flexion 110°–130° . . . . Flex knee and bring thigh close to abdomen.
Abduction 45° . . . . Swing thigh away from midline.
Adduction 30° . . . . Bring thigh toward and across the midline.
External rotation 45° . . . . Flex knee. Swing lower leg toward midline.
Internal rotation 40° . . . . Flex knee. Swing lower leg away from midline.
Knee
Extension 5°–10° beyond 180° . . . . Straighten out knee as much as possible.
Flexion 160° . . . . Touch calf to hamstring.
Ankle
Extension (Dorsiflexion) 20° . . . . Bend ankle so toes point up.
Flexion (Plantar flexion) 45° . . . . Bend ankle so toes point down.
Eversion 20° . . . . Turn foot so the sole faces out.
Inversion 30° . . . . Turn foot so the sole faces in.

Bibliography

Alter, M. J. 1996. *Science of Flexibility*. Champaign, IL: Human Kinetics.

American College of Sports Medicine. 1998. Position Stand. Exercise and physical activity for older adults. *Medicine and Science in Sports and Exercise* vol. 30, no. 6, pp. 992–1008.

Arnheim, D. D. 1986. *Dance Injuries: Their prevention and care*. Republished 1988 by Princeton Book Company, Publishers, Princeton, NJ. Originally published by C. V. Mosby Company.

Bak, K., and S. P. Magnusson. 1997. Shoulder strength and range of motion in symptomatic and pain-free elite swimmers. *American Journal of Sports Medicine* vol. 25, no. 4, pp. 454–459.

Bandy, W. D., and J. M. Irion. 1994. The effect of time of static stretch on the flexibility of the hamstring muscles. *Physical Therapy* vol. 74, no. 9, pp. 845–850.

Bandy, W. D., J. M. Irion, and M. Briggler. 1997. The effect of time and frequency of static stretching on flexibility of the hamstring muscles. *Physical Therapy* vol. 77, no. 10, pp. 1090–1096.

Bandy, W. D., J. M. Irion, and M. Briggler. 1998. The effect of static stretch and dynamic range of motion training on the flexibility of the hamstring muscles. *Journal of Orthopaedic and Sports Physical Therapy* vol. 27, no. 4, pp. 295–300.

Barbosa, A. R., J. M. Santarém, W. J. Filho, and M. N. Marucci. 2002. Effects of resistance training on the sit-and-reach test in elderly women. *Journal of Strength and Conditioning Research* vol. 16, no. 1, pp. 14–18.

Bassey, E. J., K. Morgan, H. M. Dallosso, and S. B. Ebrahim. 1989. Flexibility of the shoulder joint measured as range of abduction in a large representative sample of men and women over 65 years of age. *European Journal of Applied Physiology and Occupational Physiology* vol. 58, no. 4, pp. 353–60.

Beighton, P., R. Grahame, and H. Bird. 1983. *Hypermobility of joints*. Berlin: Springer-Verlag.

Bishop, B. 1982. *Basic Neurophysiology*. Garden City, NY: Medical Examination Publishing Co.

Borowiec, S., and A. Ronikier. 1977. *Zarys anatomii funkcjonalnej narzadow ruchu*. Warszawa: WAWF.

191

Breit, N. J. 1977. The effects of body position and stretching technique on development of hip and back flexibility. Dissertation for degree of Doctor of Physical Education. Springfield College.

Brown, M., D. R. Sinacore, A. A. Ehsani, E. F. Binder, J. O. Holloszy, and W. M. Kohrt. 2000. Low-intensity exercise as a modifier of physical frailty in older adults. *Archives of Physical Medicine and Rehabilitation* vol. 81, no. 7, pp. 960–965.

Buckwalter, J. A. 1997. Maintaining and restoring mobility in middle and old age: the importance of soft tissues. *Instructional Course Lectures* vol. 46, pp. 459–469.

Burkett, L. N. 1970. Causative factors in hamstring strains. *Medicine and Science in Sports* vol. 2, no. 1, pp. 39–42.

Chang, D. E., L. P. Buschbacher, and R. F. Edlich. 1988. Limited joint mobility in power lifters. *American Journal of Sports Medicine* vol. 16, no. 3, pp. 280–284.

Chleboun, G. S., J. N. Howell, R. R. Conatser, and J. J. Giesey. 1997. The relationship between elbow flexor volume and angular stiffness at the elbow. *Clinical Biomechanics* vol. 12, no. 6, pp. 383–392.

Ciszek, B., and R. Smigielski. 1997. *Anatomiczne zaleznosci pomiedzy strukturami kostnymi i wiezadlowymi podczas ruchow w stawach biodrowym i ramiennym.* Island Pond, VT: Stadion Publishing Co., Inc. Electronic files.

Ciullo, J. V., and B. Zarins. 1983. Biomechanics of the musculotendinous unit: relation to athletic performance and injury. *Clinics in Sports Medicine* vol. 2, no. 1, pp. 71–86.

Clarkson, P. M., K. Nosaka, and B. Braun. 1992. Muscle function after exercise-induced muscle damage and rapid adaptation. *Medicine and Science in Sports and Exercise* vol. 24, no. 5, pp. 512–520.

Craib, M. W., V. A. Mitchell, K. B. Fields, T. R. Cooper, R. Hopewell, and D. W. Morgan. 1996. The association between flexibility and running economy in sub-elite distance runners. *Medicine and Science in Sports and Exercise* vol. 28, no. 6, 737–743.

deVries, H. A. 1961. Electromyographic observations of the effects of static stretching upon muscular distress. *Research Quarterly* vol. 32, no. 4, pp. 468–479.

deVries, H. A. 1980. *Physiology of Exercise for Physical Education and Athletics.* Dubuque, IA: Wm. C. Brown Company Publishers.

Dintiman, G. B. 1964. Effects of various training programs on running speed. *Research Quarterly* vol. 35, no. 4, pp. 456–463.

Drabik, J. 1996. *Children and Sports Training: How Your Future Champions Should Exercise to Be Healthy, Fit, and Happy.* Island Pond, VT: Stadion Publishing Co., Inc.

Editors of *Georgia Tech Sports Medicine & Performance Newsletter* 1999. Stretching Machines. *Georgia Tech Sports Medicine & Performance Newsletter* vol. 7, no. 12, p. 6.

Ellison, J. B., S. J. Rose, and S. A. Sahrmann. 1990. Patterns of hip rotation range of motion: a comparison between healthy subjects and patients with low back pain. *Physical Therapy* vol. 70, no. 9, pp. 537–541.

Enoka, R. M., R. S. Hutton, and E. Eldred. 1980. Changes in excitability of tendon tap and Hoffman reflexes following voluntary contractions. *Electroencephalography and Clinical Neurophysiology* vol. 48, no. 6, pp. 664–672.

Etnyre, B. R., and L. D. Abraham. 1986a. Gains in range of ankle dorsiflexion using three popular stretching techniques. *American Journal of Physical Medicine* vol. 65, no. 4, pp. 189–196.

Etnyre, B. R. and L. D. Abraham. 1986b. H-reflex changes during static stretching and two variations of proprioceptive neuromuscular facilitation techniques. *Electroencephalography and Clinical Neurophysiology* vol. 63, no. 2, pp. 174–179.

Etnyre, B. R. and L. D. Abraham. 1988. Antagonist muscle activity during stretching: a paradox re-assessed. *Medicine and Science in Sports and Exercise* vol. 20, no. 3, pp. 285–289.

Evans, W. J. 1999. Exercise training guidelines for the elderly. *Medicine and Science in Sports and Exercise* vol. 31, no. 1, pp. 12–17.

Feiring, D. C., and G. L. Derscheid. 1989. The role of preseason conditioning in preventing athletic injuries. *Clinics in Sports Medicine* vol. 8, no. 3, pp. 361–372.

Feldman, D., I. Shrier, M. Rossignol, and L. Abenhaim. 1999. Adolescent growth is not associated with changes in flexibility. *Clinical Journal of Sport Medicine* vol. 9, no. 1, pp. 24–29.

Fiatarone, M. A., E. C. Marks, N. D. Ryan, C. N. Meredith, L. A. Lipsitz, and W. J. Evans. 1990. High-intensity strength training in nonagenarians. Effects on skeletal muscle. *JAMA* vol. 263, no. 22, pp. 3029–3034.

Fleisig, G. S. Andrews, J. R., Dillman, C. J., and Escamilla, R. F. 1995. Kinetics of baseball pitching with implication about injury mechanisms. *American Journal of Sports Medicine* vol. 23, no. 2, pp. 233–239.

Fowles, J. R., D. G. Sale, and J. D. MacDougall. 2000. Reduced strength after passive stretch of the human plantarflexors. *Journal of Applied Physiology* vol. 89, no. 3, pp. 1179–1188.

Fox, E. L. 1979. *Sports Physiology*. Philadelphia: Saunders College Publishing.

Fridén, J. 1984. Changes in human skeletal muscle induced by long-term eccentric exercise. *Cell and Tissue Research* vol. 236, no. 2, pp. 365–372.

Fridén, J., and R. L. Lieber. 1992. Structural and mechanical basis of exercise-induced muscle injury. *Medicine and Science in Sports and Exercise* vol. 24, no. 5, pp. 521–530.

Garrett, W. E., Jr. 1996. Muscle strain injuries. *American Journal of Sports Medicine* vol. 24, no. 6 Supplement, pp. S2–S8.

Gersten, J. W. 1991. Effect of exercise on muscle function decline with aging. *The Western Journal of Medicine* vol. 154, no. 4, pp. 579–582.

Geselevich, V. A. 1976. *Meditsinskiy spravochnik trenera*. Moscow: Fizkultura i Sport.

Girouard, C. K., and B. F. Hurley. 1995. Does strength training inhibit gains in range of motion from flexibility training in older adults? *Medicine and Science in Sports and Exercise* vol. 27, no. 10, pp. 1444–1449.

Gleim, G. W., and M. P. McHugh. 1997. Flexibility and its effects on sports injury and performance. *Sports Medicine* vol. 24, no. 5, pp. 289–299.

Goldspink, G. 1968. Sarcomere length during post-natal growth of mammalian muscle fibres. *Journal of Cell Science* vol. 3, no. 4, pp. 539–548.

Grochmal, S. 1986. *Teoria i metodyka cwiczen relaksowo-koncentrujacych.* Warsaw: PZWL.

Growdon, W., J. Ghika, J. Henderson, G. van Melle, F. Regli, J. Bogousslavsky, and J. H. Growdon. 2000. Effects of proximal and distal muscles' groups contraction and mental stress on the amplitude and frequency of physical finger tremor. An accelerometric study. *Electromyography and Clinical Neurophysiology* vol. 40, no. 5, pp. 295–303.

Gullich, A., and D. Schmidtbleicher. 1996. MVC-induced short-term potentiation of explosive force. *New Studies in Athletics* vol. 4. pp. 67–81. Quoted in W. Young and S. Elliott. 2001. Acute effects of static stretching, proprioceptive neuromuscular facilitation stretching, and maximal voluntary contractions on explosive force production and jumping performance. *Research Quarterly for Exercise and Sport* vol. 72, no. 3, pp. 273–279.

Halbertsma, J. P., and L. N. Goeken. 1994. Stretching exercises: effect on passive extensibility and stiffness in short hamstrings of healthy subjects. *Archives of Physical Medicine and Rehabilitation* vol. 75, no. 9, pp. 976–981.

Halbertsma, J. P., A. I. van Bolhuis, and L. N. Goeken. 1996. Sport stretching: effect on passive muscle stiffness of short hamstrings. *Archives of Physical Medicine and Rehabilitation* vol. 77, no. 7, pp. 688–692.

Handel, M., T. Horstmann, H. H. Dickhuth, and R. W. Gulch. 1997. Effects of contract-relaxed stretching training on muscle performance in athletes. *European Journal of Applied Physiology and Occupational Physiology* vol. 76. no. 5, pp. 400–408.

Hartig, D. E., and J. M. Henderson. 1999. Increasing hamstring flexibility decreases lower extremity overuse injuries in military basic trainees. *American Journal of Sports Medicine* vol. 27, no. 2, 173–176.

Harvey, J. and S. Tanner. 1991. Low back pain in young athletes. A practical approach. *Sports Medicine* vol. 12, no. 6, pp. 394–406.

Hayes, K. C. 1976. A Theory of the Mechanism of Muscular Strength Development Upon EMG Evidence of Motor Unit Synchronization. In *Biomechanics of Sports and Kinanthropometry,* ed. F. Landry and W. A. R. Orban. pp. 69–77. Miami, FL: Symposia Specialists, Inc.

Hertling, D. and R. M. Kessler. 1996. *Management of Common Musculoskeletal Disorders: Physical Therapy Principles and Methods.* Philadelphia: Lippincott Williams & Wilkins.

Hettinger, T., and E. A. Müller. 1953. Muskelleistung und Muskeltraining. *Arbeitsphysiologie* vol. 15, pp. 111–126. Quoted in H. A. deVries, *Physiology of Exercise for Physical Education and Athletics.* (Dubuque, IA: Wm. C. Brown Company Publishers, 1980).

Holt, L. E., T. M. Travis, and T. Okita. 1970. Comparative study of three stretching techniques. *Perceptual and Motor Skills* vol. 31, no. 2, pp. 611–616.

Houk, J. C., J. J. Singer, and E. Henneman. 1971. Adequate stimulus for tendon organs with observations on mechanics of ankle joint. *Journal of Neurophysiology* vol. 34, no. 6, pp. 1051–1065.

Howell, D. W. 1984. Musculoskeletal profile and incidence of musculoskeletal injuries in lightweight women rowers. *American Journal of Sports Medicine* vol. 12, no. 4, pp. 278–282.

James, B., and A. W. Parker. 1989. Active and passive mobility of lower limb joints in elderly men and women. *American Journal of Physical Medicine and Rehabilitation* vol. 68, no. 4, pp. 162–167.

Johansson, P. H., L. Lindstrom, G. Sundelin, and B. Lindstrom. 1999. The effects of preexercise stretching on muscular soreness, tenderness and force loss following heavy eccentric exercise. *Scandinavian Journal of Medicine and Science in Sports* vol. 9, no. 4, pp. 219–225.

Kapandji, I. A. 1982. *The Physiology of the Joints. Volume One: Upper Limb.* Edinburgh: Churchill Livingstone.

Kapandji, I. A. 1987. *The Physiology of the Joints. Volume Two: Lower Limb.* Edinburgh: Churchill Livingstone.

Kapandji, I. A. 1974. *The Physiology of the Joints. Volume Three: The Trunk and the Vertebral Column.* Edinburgh: Churchill Livingstone.

Kirby, R. L., F. C. Simms, V. J. Symington, and J. B. Garner. 1981. Flexibility and musculoskeletal symptomatology in female gymnasts and age-matched controls. *American Journal of Sports Medicine* vol. 9, no. 3, pp. 160–164.

Klinge, K., S. P. Magnusson, E. B. Simonsen, P. Aagaard, K. Klausen, and M. Kjaer. 1997. The effect of strength and flexibility training on skeletal muscle electromyographic activity, stiffness, and viscoelastic stress relaxation response. *American Journal of Sports Medicine* vol. 25, no. 5, pp. 710–716.

Knapik, J. J., C. L. Bauman, B. H. Jones, J. M. Harris, and L. Vaughan. 1991. Preseason strength and flexibility imbalances associated with athletic injuries in female collegiate athletes. *American Journal of Sports Medicine* vol. 19, no. 1, pp. 76–81.

Kokkonen, J., A. G. Nelson and A. Cornwell. 1998. Acute muscle stretching inhibits maximal strength performance. *Research Quarterly for Exercise and Sport* vol. 69, no. 4, pp. 411–415.

Kokkonen, J., and S. Lauritzen. 1995. Isotonic strength and endurance gains through PNF stretching. *Medicine and Science in Sports and Exercise* vol. 27, no. 5, p. S22.

Koslow, R. E. 1987. Bilateral flexibility in the upper and lower extremities as related to age and gender. *Journal of Human Movement Studies* vol. 13, no. 9, pp. 467–472.

Krivickas, L. S. 1997. Anatomical factors associated with overuse sports injuries. *Sports Medicine* vol. 24, no. 2, pp. 132–146.

Krivickas, L. S., and J. H. Feinberg. 1996. Lower extremity injuries in college athletes: relation between ligamentous laxity and lower extremity muscle tightness. *Archives of Physical Medicine and Rehabilitation* vol. 77, no. 11, pp. 1139–1143.

Kubo, K., Y. Kawakami, and T. Fukunaga. 1999. Influence of elastic properties of tendon structures on jump performance in humans. *Journal of Applied Physiology* vol. 87, no. 6, pp. 2090–2096.)

Kubo, K., H. Kanehisa, and T. Fukunaga. 2001a. Effects of different duration isometric contractions on tendon elasticity in human quadriceps muscles. *Journal of Physiology* vol. 15, no. 536, pp. 649–655.

Kubo, K., H. Kanehisa, M. Ito, and T. Fukunaga. 2001b. Effects of isometric training on the elasticity of human tendon in vivo. *Journal of Applied Physiology* vol. 91, no. 1, pp. 26–32.

Kubo, K., H. Kanehisa, and T. Fukunaga. 2002a. Effects of resistance and stretching training programmes on the viscoelastic properties of human tendon structures in vivo. *Journal of Physiology* vol. 538, pp. 219–226.

Kubo, K., H. Kanehisa, and T. Fukunaga. 2002b. Effect of stretching training on the viscoelastic properties of human tendon structures in vivo. *Journal of Applied Physiology* vol. 92, no. 2, pp. 595–601.

Kushner, S., L. Saboe, D. Reid, T. Penrose, M. Grace. 1990. Relationship of turnout to hip abduction in professional ballet dancers. *American Journal of Sports Medicine* vol. 18, no. 3, pp. 286–291.

Lazowski, D. A., N. A. Ecclestone, A .M. Myers, D. H. Patterson, C. Tudor -Locke, C. Fitzgerald, G. Jones, N. Shima, and D. A. Cunningham. 1999. A randomized outcome evaluation of group exercise programs in long-term care institutions. *The Journals of Gerontology. Series A, Biological Sciences and Medical Sciences.* vol. 54, no. 12, pp. M621–628.

Lexell, J., D. Y. Downham, Y. Larsson, E. Bruhn, and B. Morsing. 1995. Heavy resistance training in older Scandinavian men and women: short- and long-term effects on arm and leg muscles. *Scandinavian Journal of Medicine and Science in Sports* vol. 5, no. 6, pp. 329–341.

Lieber, R. L., and J. Fridén. 2000. Functional and clinical significance of skeletal muscle architecture. *Muscle and Nerve* vol. 23, no. 11, pp. 1647–1666.

Logan, G. A., and G. H. Egstrom. 1961. Effects of slow and fast stretching on the sacrofemoral angle. *Journal of the Association for Physical and Mental Rehabilitation* vol. 15, no. 3, pp. 85–89.

Logan, G. A., and W. C. McKinney. 1970. *Kinesiology.* Dubuque, IA: Wm. C. Brown Company Publishers.

Lucas, R. C. and R. Koslow. 1984. Comparative study of static, dynamic, and proprioceptive neuromuscular facilitation stretching techniques on flexibility. *Perceptual and Motor Skills* vol. 58, no. 2, pp. 615–618.

Magnusson, S. P., E. B. Simonsen, P. Aagaard, P. Dyhre-Poulsen, M. P. McHugh, and M. Kjaer. 1996a. Mechanical and physical responses to stretching with and without preisometric contraction in human skeletal muscle. *Archives of Physical Medicine and Rehabilitation* vol. 77, no. 4, pp. 373–378.

Magnusson, S. P., E. B. Simonsen, P. Aagaard, H. Sorensen, and M. Kjaer. 1996b. A mechanism for altered flexibility in human skeletal muscle. *Journal of Physiology* vol. 497, pp. 291–298.

Magnusson, S. P., E. B. Simonsen, P. Aagaard, J. Boesen, F. Johannsen, and M. Kjaer. 1997. Determinants of musculoskeletal flexibility: viscoelastic properties, cross-sectional area, EMG and stretch tolerance. *Scandinavian Journal of Medicine and Science in Sports* vol. 7, no. 4, pp. 195–202.

Magnusson, S. P., P. Aagaard, E. Simonsen, and F. Bojsen-Moller. 1998. A biomechanical evaluation of cyclic and static stretch in human skeletal muscle. *International Journal of Sports Medicine* vol. 19, no. 5, pp. 310–316.

Marciniak, J. 1991. *Zbior cwiczen koordynacyjnych i gibkosciowych.* Warszawa: RCMSKFiS.

Matveyev, L. P. [Matveev, L. P.] 1981. *Fundamentals of Sports Training.* Moscow: Progress Publishers.

McArdle, W. D., F. I. Katch, and V. L. Katch. 1996. *Exercise Physiology: Energy, Nutrition, and Human Performance.* Baltimore: Williams & Wilkins.

McHugh, M. P., I. J. Kremenic, M. B. Fox, G. W. Gleim. 1998. The role of mechanical and neural restraints to joint range of motion during passive stretch. *Medicine and Science in Sports and Exercise* vol. 30, no. 6, pp. 928–932.

McMaster, W. C., S. C. Long, and V. J. Caiozzo. 1991. Isokinetic torque imbalances in the rotator cuff of the elite water polo player. *The American Journal of Sports Medicine* vol. 19, no. 1, pp. 72–75.

McMaster, W. C., A. Roberts, and T. Stoddard. 1998. A correlation between shoulder laxity and interfering pain in competitive swimmers. *American Journal of Sports Medicine* vol. 26, no. 1, pp. 83–86.

McMaster, W. C., and J. Troup. 1993. A survey of interfering shoulder pain in United States competitive swimmers. *American Journal of Sports Medicine* vol. 21, no. 1, pp. 67–70.

McNair, P. J., and S. N. Stanley. 1996. Effect of passive stretching and jogging on the series elastic muscle stiffness and range of motion of the ankle joint. *British Journal of Sports Medicine* vol. 30, no. 4, pp. 313–318.

McNair, P. J., E. W. Dombroski, D. J. Hewson, and S. N. Stanley. 2001. Stretching at the ankle joint: viscoelastic responses to holds and continuous passive motion. *Medicine and Science in Sports and Exercise* vol. 33, no. 3, pp. 354–358.

Meeusen, R., and P. Lievens. 1986. The use of cryotherapy in sports injuries. *Sports Medicine* vol. 3, no. 6, pp. 398–414.

Micheli, L. J. 1990. *Sportswise: An Essential Guide for Young Athletes, Parents, and Coaches.* Boston: Houghton Mifflin Company.

Miles, M. P., and P. M. Clarkson. 1994. Exercise-induced muscle pain, soreness, and cramps. *Journal of Sports Medicine and Physical Fitness* vol. 34, no. 3, pp. 203–216.

Moller, M. H., B. E. Oberg, and J. Gillquist. 1985. Stretching exercise and soccer: effect of stretching on range of motion in the lower extremity in connection with soccer training. *International Journal of Sports Medicine* vol. 6, no. 1, pp. 50–52.

Moore, M. A., and C. G. Kukulka. 1991. Depression of Hoffman reflexes following voluntary contraction and implications for proprioceptive neuromuscular facilitation therapy. *Physical Therapy* vol. 71, no. 4, pp. 321–329.

Morgan, K. A. 2000. The effects of acute muscle stretching on maximal muscle performance. Master's thesis, Eastern Michigan University.

Moritani, T., and H. A. deVries. 1979. Neural factors versus hypertrophy in the time course of muscle strength gain. *American Journal of Physical Medicine* vol. 58, no. 3, pp. 115–130.

Moscov, J., and M. G. Lacourse. 1992. Static range of motion, leg power, and leg strength as predictors of dynamic range of motion in female ballet dancers. *Research Quarterly Exercise and Sport* vol. 63, no. 1, Supplement pp. A-19–A-24.

Murphy, D. R. 1991. A critical look at static stretching: are we doing our patients harm? *Chiropractic Sports Medicine* vol. 5, no. 3, pp. 67–70.

Müller, E. A., and W. Röhmert. 1963. Die Geschwindigkeit der Muskelkraft—Zunahme bei isometrischen Training. *Arbeitsphysiologie* vol. 19, pp. 403–419. Quoted in H. A. deVries, *Physiology of Exercise for Physical Education and Athletics.* (Dubuque, IA: Wm. C. Brown Company Publishers, 1980).

Nelson, K. C., and W. L. Cornelius. 1991. The relationship between isometric contraction durations and improvement in shoulder joint range of motion. *Journal of Sports Medicine and Physical Fitness* vol. 31, no. 3, pp. 385–388.

Nelson, A. G. and J. Kokkonen. 2001. Acute Ballistic Muscle Stretching Inhibits Maximal Strength Performance. Research *Quarterly for Exercise and Sport* vol. 72, no. 4, pp. 415–419.

Orchard, J., J. Marsden, S. Lord, and D. Garlick 1997. Preseason hamstring muscle weakness associated with hamstring muscle injury in Australian footballers. *American Journal of Sports Medicine* vol. 25, no. 1, pp. 81–85.

Orlikowska, A. 1991. Zastosowanie poizometrycznej relaksacji miesni i stretchingu w odnowie biologicznej sportowcow. In *W kregu psychofizykalnych zagadnien profilaktyki i terapii w sporcie,* ed. W. Tlokinski, pp. 9–22. Gdansk: AWF.

Ozolin, N. G. 1971. *Sovermennaya systema sportivnoy trenirovki.* Moscow: Fizkultura i Sport. Quoted in T. O. Bompa, *Periodization: Theory and Methodology of Training.* (Champaign, IL: Human Kinetics, 1999), pp. 48, 380.)

Pappas, A. M., R. M. Zawacki, and C. F. McCarthy. 1985. Rehabilitation of the pitching shoulder. *American Journal of Sports Medicine* vol. 13, no. 4, pp. 223–235.

Platonov, V. N. 1997. *Obshchaya teoriya podgotovki sportsmenov v olimpiyskom sporte.* Kiev: Olimpiyskaya Literatura.

Platonov, V. N., and S. L. Fesenko. 1990. *Silneyshe plovcy mira.* Moscow: Fizkultura i Sport.

Ploutz, L. L., P. A. Tesch, R. L. Biro, and G. A. Dudley. 1994. Effect of resistance training on muscle use during exercise. *Journal of Applied Physiology* vol. 76, no. 4, pp. 1675–1681.

Pope, R. P., R. D. Herbert, J. D. Kirvan, and B. J. Graham. 2000. A randomized trial of preexercise stretching for prevention of lower-limb injury. *Medicine and Science in Sports and Exercise* vol. 32, no. 2, pp. 271–277.

Potter, P. A. 1986. *Pocket Nurse Guide to Physical Assessment.* St. Louis: The C. V. Mosby Company.

Raczek, J. 1991. *Podstawy szkolenia sportowego dzieci i mlodziezy.* Warsaw: RCMSKFiS.

Reid, D. C. 1988. Prevention of hip and knee injuries in ballet dancers. *Sports Medicine* vol. 6, no. 5, pp. 295–307.

Reid, D. A. and P. J. McNair. 2000. Factors contributing to low back pain in rowers. *British Journal of Sports Medicine* vol. 34, no. 5, pp. 321–322.

Reid, D. C., R. S. Burnham, L. A. Saboe, and S. F. Kushner. 1987. Lower extremity flexibility patterns in classical ballet dancers and their correlation to lateral hip and knee injuries. *American Journal of Sports Medicine* vol. 15, no. 4, pp. 347–352.

Renström, P. and R. J. Johnson. 1986. Presentation at Second Scandinavian Conference in Sports Medicine. Quoted in Editors of *Sport Wyczynowy*. 1994. Urazy z przeciazenia—wielki problem sportu. *Sport Wyczynowy* no. 3–4/351–352, pp. 63–72.

Repice, F., L. Iannucci, R. Lepri, G., Magnolfi, A. Malacarne, M. Mancini, L. Mori, and C. J. Giannini. 1982. Osservazioni sui rapporti esistenti tra tipo constituzionale e motilità articolare. Parte II. *Archivio Italiano di Anatomia e di Embriologia* vol. 87, no. 4, pp. 301–313.

Roberts, J. M., and K. Wilson. 1999. Effect of stretching duration on active and passive range of motion in the lower extremity. *British Journal of Sports Medicine* vol. 33, no. 4, pp. 259–263.

Rosenbaum, D., and E. M. Hennig. 1995. The influence of stretching and warm-up exercises on Achilles tendon reflex activity. *Journal of Sport Sciences* vol. 13, no. 6, pp. 481–490.

Rudy, D. M. 1987. The relationship of fatigability and flexibility to hamstring injuries in sprinters. *Medicine and Science in Sports and Exercise* vol. 19, no. 2 Supplement. Quoted in Editors of *Sport Wyczynowy*. 1987. Przeglad Literatury. *Sport Wyczynowy* no. 12/276 (1987), pp. 63–66.

Ryan, A. J. and R. E. Stephens. 1988. *The Dancer's Complete Guide to Healthcare and a Long Career.* Princeton, NJ: Princeton Book Company, Publishers.

Sady, S. P., M. Wortman, and D. Blanke. 1982. Flexibility training: ballistic, static or proprioceptive neuromuscular facilitation? *Archives of Physical Medicine and Rehabilitation* vol. 63, no. 6, pp. 261–263.

Safran, M. R., A. V. Seaber, and W. E. Garrett Jr. 1989. Warm-up and muscular injury prevention. An update. *Sports Medicine* vol. 8, no. 4, pp. 239–249.

Sandstead, H. L. 1968. The relationship of outward rotation of the humerus to baseball throwing velocity. Master's thesis, Eastern Illinois University, Charleston.

Saxton, J. M., and A. E. Donnelly. 1996. Length-specific impairment of skeletal muscle contractile function after eccentric muscle actions in man. *Clinical Science* vol. 90, no. 2, pp. 119–125.

Schottelius, B. A., and L. C. Senay. 1956. Effect of stimulation-length sequence on shape of length-tension diagram. *American Journal of Physiology* vol. 186, no. 1, pp. 127–130.

Sermeev, B. V. 1968. Razvitie podvizhnosti u legkoatletov. Legkaya Atletika no. 9, p. 13.

Shrier, I. 1999. Stretching before exercise does not reduce the risk of local muscle injury: a critical review of the clinical and basic science literature. *Clinical Journal of Sport Medicine* vol. 9, no. 4, pp. 221–227.

Shrier, I. 2000. Stretching before exercise: an evidence based approach. *British Journal of Sports Medicine* vol. 34, no. 5, pp. 324–325.

Siff, M. C., and Y. V. Verkhoshansky. 1999. *Supertraining*. Denver, CO: Supertraining International.

Smith, L. L., M. H. Brunetz, T. C. Chenier, M. R. McCammon, J. A. Houmard, M. E. Franklin, R. G. Israel. 1993. The effects of static and ballistic stretching on delayed onset muscle soreness and creatine kinase. *Research Quarterly for Exercise and Sport* vol. 64, no. 1, pp. 103–107.

Sölveborn, S. A. 1989. *Stretching*. Warsaw: Sport i Turystyka.

Starzynski, T. and H. Sozanski. 1999. *Explosive Power and Jumping Ability for All Sports: Atlas of Exercises*. Island Pond, VT: Stadion Publishing Co. Inc.

Strzelczyk, P. 1996. Krioterapia w leczeniu i rehabilitacji urazow sportowych. *Sport Wyczynowy* no. 11–12/383–384, pp. 107–113.

Tanigawa, M. C. 1972. Comparison of the hold-relax procedure and passive mobilization on increasing muscle length. *Physical Therapy* vol. 52, no. 7, pp. 725–735.

Tipton, C. M., R. D. Matthes, J. A. Maynard, and R. A. Carey. 1975. The influence of physical activity on ligaments and tendons. *Medicine and Science in Sports* vol. 7, no. 3, pp. 165–175.

Toft, E., G. T. Espersen, S. Kalund, T. Sinkjaer, and B. C. Hornemann. 1989. Passive tension of the ankle before and after stretching. *American Journal of Sports Medicine* vol. 17, no. 4, pp. 489–494.

Tumanyan, G. S., and Sh. M. Dzhanyan. 1980. Strength exercises as a means of improving active flexibility of wrestlers. *Teoriya i Praktika Fizicheskoy Kultury* no. 10, pp. 10–11. In *Soviet Sports Review* vol. 19, no. 3 (September 1984), pp. 146–150.

Tumanyan, G. S., and S. K. Kharatsidis. 1998. Gibkost' kak fizicheskoye kachestvo. *Teorya i Praktika Fizicheskoy Kultury* no. 2, pp. 48–50.

Tyler, T. F., S. J. Nicholas, R. J. Campbell, and M. P. McHugh. 2001. The association of hip strength and flexibility with the incidence of adductor muscle strains in professional ice hockey players. *American Journal of Sports Medicine* vol. 29, no. 2, pp. 124–128.

Vander, A. J. J. H. Sherman, and D. S. Luciano. 2001. *Human Physiology—The Mechanisms of Body Function*. New York: McGraw-Hill.

Wallin, D., B. Ekblom, R. Grahn, and T. Nordenborg. 1985. Improvement of muscle flexibility. A comparison between two techniques. *American Journal of Sports Medicine* vol. 13, no. 4, pp. 263–268.

Walther, D. S. 2000. *Applied Kinesiology: Synopsis*. Pueblo, CO: Systems DC.

Wazny, Z. 1981a. Koordynacja ruchowa. In *Teoria i metodyka sportu*, ed. T. Ulatowski, pp. 156–164. Warsaw: Sport i Turystyka.

Wazny, Z. 1981b. Gibkosc. In *Teoria i metodyka sportu*, ed. T. Ulatowski, pp. 165–170. Warsaw: Sport i Turystyka.

Williams P. E., T. Catanese, E. G. Lucey, and G. Goldspink. 1988. The importance of stretch and contractile activity in the prevention of connective tissue accumulation in muscle. *Journal of Anatomy* no. 158, pp. 109–114.

Williford, H. N., J. B. East, F. H. Smith, and L. A. Burry. 1986. Evaluation of warm-up for improvement in flexibility. *American Journal of Sports Medicine* vol. 14, no. 4, pp. 316–319.

Wilmore, J. H. and D. L. Costill. 1999. *Physiology of Sport and Exercise*. Champaign, IL: Human Kinetics.

Wilson, G. J., B. C. Elliott, and G. A. Wood. 1992. Stretch shorten cycle performance enhancement through flexibility training. *Medicine and Science in Sports and Exercise* vol. 24, no. 1, pp. 116–123.

Wilson, G. J., A. J. Murphy, and J. F. Pryor. 1994. Musculotendinous stiffness: its relationship to eccentric, isometric, and concentric performance. *Journal of Applied Physiology* vol. 76, no. 6, pp. 2714–2719.

Witvrouw, E., J. Bellemans, R. Lysens, L. Danneels, and D. Cambier. 2001. Intrinsic risk factors for the development of patellar tendinitis in an athletic population. A two-year prospective study. *American Journal of Sports Medicine* vol. 29, no. 2, pp. 190–195.

Worrell, T. W., T. L. Smith, and J. Winegardner. 1994. Effect of hamstring stretching on hamstring muscle performance. *Journal of Orthopaedic and Sports Physical Therapy* vol. 20, no. 3, pp. 154–159.

Young, W., and S. Elliott. 2001. Acute effects of static stretching, proprioceptive neuromuscular facilitation stretching, and maximum voluntary contractions on explosive force production and jumping performance. *Research Quarterly for Exercise and Sport* vol. 72, no. 3, p. 273–279.

Zelisko, J. A., H. B. Noble, and M. Porter. 1982. A comparison of men's and women's professional basketball injuries. *American Journal of Sports Medicine* vol. 10, no. 5, pp. 297–299.

Standard workout layout

Aerobic warmup increasing heart rate & altering breathing
General dynamic stretches.

Term "group of muscles" doesn't mean in an area, rather
the individual group working towards the same goal. Eg hamst

Morning stretches P19

Index

A

Abdomen
  isometric stretches for, 72–73
  relaxed stretches for, 86–87
Abduction
  adductors and, 110
  hip, 174, 186, 189
  hip flexion and, 111
  shoulder, 187, 189
Acrobatics
  flexibility and, 6
Actin
  muscle cell and, 105
Active flexibility
  passive flexibility and, 49
Adduction
  hip, 189
  shoulder, 189
Adductors
  function, 110
  side split and, 128
Adolescents
  isometric stretching and, 49, 156
Advanced
  morning stretch and, 19
Age
  flexibility and, 25–27, 103, 156
  stretching and, 126, 156
Amplitude of movement
  increasing, 49
  tired muscles and, 14
  trunk and, 37
Ankle
  dorsiflexion, 189
  eversion, 189
  extension, 189
  flexion, 189
  inversion, 189
  normal range of motion, 189
  plantar flexion, 189
Anxiety
  flexibility and, 118

Applied Kinesiology
  injury and, 166
  International College of, 165
Arm swings, 5, 14, 19, 21, 33
Arms
  dynamic stretches for, 33
  isometric stretches for, 58–59
  relaxed stretches for, 79
  static active stretches for, 41

B

Back
  dynamic stretches for, 38
  extension, 48
  See also Lower back
  See also Lumbar spine
  relaxed stretches for, 86
  static active stretches for, 45
  See also Upper back
Ballet
  first position, 110
Ballistic stretches
  children and, 26
  definition, 15
Ballistic stretching
  children and, 108
  definition, 15
  static stretching and, 120
Basketball
  stretches for, 58
Beginners
  dynamic stretches, 34
  morning stretch and, 19
Bending
  lumbar spine, 189
  neck, 189
Bicycling
  flexibility and, 121
Blood flow
  flexibility and, 19, 21, 122
  stretching and, 104

203

Test Your Flexibility Potential

Will you be able to do splits after following this stretching method?

Do these tests to determine if you have the potential to do front and side splits even before you start our stretching program.

Deep lunge. The knee of the front leg is flexed and the angle between thighs is 180 degrees.

Front split test: Stand in a deep lunge. If your thighs are nearly in one line, as they should be in a front split, it means that your hip joints and their ligaments do not prevent you from doing the front split. Only tightness of your muscles may keep you from sitting in a flat front split with both legs straight. With our stretching method you will relax, or even elongate, these muscles and be able to do the front split with no warm-up.

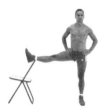

If you think that the length of your muscles and structure of your hips will not let you do side splits, try this test . . .

The leg resting on the chair is in the position it would have in a split

Side split test: Stand beside a chair or table and put your leg on it as shown below. Make sure that both your hips and your raised leg are all in one line. Repeat this test with your other leg.

Now, what have you done? You have done "half side splits" with both your legs!

You have proved to yourself that both your hip joints have all the mobility (range of motion) needed for a full side split!

You have also proved that the muscles of each of your legs are already long enough for a side split. You know that no muscle or ligament runs from one inner thigh to the other (or, if you don't know it, you can ask your doctor). So, what keeps you from doing the whole side split with both legs spread sideways at the same time? This book will tell you that and how to learn to do side splits any time, without any warm-up!